Silent Battles

THE TOUGHEST BATTLES ARE THE ONES WE FIGHT ALONE

DANESHIA DRAKEFORD

SILENT BATTLES

The toughest Battles are the ones we fight alone

Daneshia Drakeford

For permission requests, write to the publisher at:

Jacinth Media Productions

info@JacinthMediaProductions.com

ISBN-13: 978-1-960594-39-6 (Hardback)

ISBN-13: 978-1-960594-38-9 (Paperback)

ISBN-13: 978-1-960594-40-2 (E-Book)

Printed in the United States of America

Contents

Disclaimer

This book is a memoir. It reflects the author's personal memories, experiences, and interpretations of events. While every effort has been made to ensure accuracy, some names, locations, dates, and identifying details have been changed to protect the privacy of individuals.

The events are recounted as remembered by the author. Dialogue is reconstructed to the best of the author's recollection. Memories are inherently subjective, and other participants in the events may have different perspectives of what occurred.

This work is not intended to malign any person, living or dead, or to depict any institution or organization in a false or negative light. Where real names are used, the intent is solely to share the author's lived experience, not to assert objective fact or cause harm.

Dedication

I dedicate this book to my hero, my late great father, **Daniel Drakeford**. Dad, I know you would be proud of me. You always put our family first and made sure we were taken care of, lacking nothing, no matter what it cost you. Your strength, wisdom, and unwavering love continue to guide me through life's uncertainties. I can almost hear your voice telling me, *"You got this, baby girl."* As I step out on faith and finally speak my truth, I carry your legacy of resilience and selflessness in every word I write. I pray this book makes you proud.

To my charming son, **Theodore Hatwood III**, my miracle baby, you are my source of strength. You have changed me in ways I never imagined. At times, when I don't know where I find the courage, it is your resilience that reflects in me, helping me realize just how deep my own endurance runs. Through your laughter, your joy, and your spirit, I find the courage to tell my story. You, T3, are the embodiment of hope and strength, and

I promise to always honor you by being the best version of myself as your mother. T3, I will never let you down.

To my beautiful mother, **Susie Drakeford**, thank you for always reminding me that God will never leave me and that you would never leave me either. You've been my rock, my constant reminder that no matter what, God has my back. I'll never forget the dream you had of God showing you that I would always be protected and covered. You saw an airplane guiding me, and in the dream, my car became super big, just as the airplane guided me safely off the road and into the parking lot at Home Depot. Your faith and vision have always been a source of strength for me. Thank you for always helping me stay anchored in my spirituality and for teaching me to maintain my relationship with God first and foremost.

To my immediate siblings **Dwight Drakeford, Syrinthia (Renny) Blount, April Drakeford** and **loved ones**, your support, love, and presence, whether loud or silent, have carried me more than you know. Also, to my two nephews, **Scott & Jaylen,** and my great-niece **Leah,** who continue to bring joy and light into my life. To my late great cousin, **Andre aka bubba.** We love and miss you so much. Thank all you for holding space for me, cheering for me, and loving me in every version of myself. This book belongs to all of you too.

Lastly, this book is also dedicated to the **warriors of the Multiple Sclerosis community**. You are the quiet strength the world doesn't always see. Living with MS means waking up to a different body every day, facing unknowns, and fighting battles most people can't imagine. As we know, living with MS comes with so many uncertainties. No two MS journeys are the same, yet we all carry this disease in our own way. We walk this journey differently, but we carry an invisible bond. You inspire me. You remind me I'm not alone. May these pages bring you peace, comfort, solidarity, and a reminder that your fight is valid. You are not weak; you are warriors.

And finally, always remember: We have MS; MS does not have us.

This isn't just *my* story.
It's *your* story.
It's *our* story.

And these are our Silent Battles.

Introduction

We all have a story that people don't see. It's the story that plays out in the quiet moments after the kids are in bed, in the car on the way to work, in the middle of the night when you're staring at the ceiling, wondering how you're going to get through tomorrow. It's the story whispered in prayers, screamed into pillows, and held tightly in the deepest parts of our hearts. It's the story of our silent battles.

For nearly twenty years, my silent battle had a name: Multiple Sclerosis. But it also had other names: fear, uncertainty, shame, and loneliness. For most of my life, I lived with this secret tucked away, hidden behind a bright smile and a "keep it pushing" attitude. I was a daughter, a sister, a wife, a mother, an actress, an employee. I wore a hundred different hats, and I was determined to wear them all perfectly, terrified that if anyone saw the cracks, if they knew the truth of what it took for me to just get through a day, they would see me as broken. As a handicap. As less than.

I thought being strong meant being silent. I thought it meant never letting anyone see the struggle, never admitting that I was tired, scared, or in pain. I spent years building walls around my heart, convinced that vulnerability was a weakness I couldn't afford.

This book is the sound of those walls coming down.

What you are about to read is not just a story about living with a chronic illness. It is a story about what happens when life, in its brutal and beautiful way, forces you to face the truths you've been running from. It's a story about a marriage that was supposed to be a safe harbor but became its own kind of storm. It's a story about the profound, all-consuming, and sometimes terrifying journey of motherhood. It's a story about becoming a caregiver for my own mother, watching the strongest woman I knew slowly fade, all while I was fighting my own battles. It's a story about hitting rock bottom, about standing in the wreckage of a life I thought I wanted, and finding the courage to start over.

I didn't write this book because I have all the answers. I wrote it because, for a long time, I had nothing but questions. I wrote it because I know what it feels like to be fighting a war that no one else can see, to feel completely and utterly alone in your struggle. I wrote it because I finally realized that my silence wasn't protecting me; it was isolating me. My secret wasn't my shield; it was my cage.

This is the story of how I found my way out of that cage. It's messy, it's raw, and it's not always pretty. There are moments of deep pain, doubt, and heartbreak. But there are also moments of unexpected grace, fierce love, and a resilience I never knew I possessed. It is the story of how I learned that true strength isn't about never falling; it's about how you choose to get back up. It's about learning to be your own hero, even when you're scared.

We all fight battles that the world knows nothing about. Maybe yours is an illness, a broken heart, a secret grief, or a dream you're afraid to chase. Whatever your silent battle may be, I want you to know this: you are not alone. My hope is that in sharing my story, in laying my own battles bare, you might find a piece of your own story reflected in these pages. I hope you find the courage to speak your own truth, even if it's just to yourself at first. And most of all, I hope you are reminded of the incredible, unbreakable strength that lies within you, waiting to be unleashed.

This is my story.

This is my battle.

And this is my truth.

Chapter 1

OUT OF NOWHERE

Before my life got complicated, it was just... normal. And normal was good. I was in my twenties, juggling a million and one things, bursting with energy. I spent my days attending college classes for my theatre degree and working at Home Depot, where I had just been promoted to a head cashier. I was proud of that. I had my own car, a healthy and fun dating life, and a sense that I was building something—brick by brick—that belonged only to me.

I never thought twice about my health. Why would I? It was reliable. Unremarkable. I was living a normal life with a healthy body that carried me through long days and late nights.

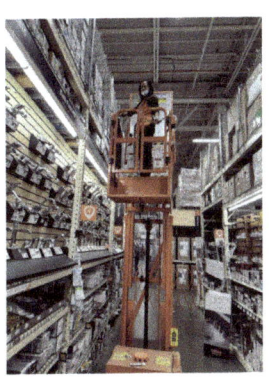

Until the day it betrayed me.

It started on the highway. I was in my red sports car, my baby, the second nice car that I bought for myself, on my way to a shift at Home Depot. The windows were down, I was blasting house music, and just enjoying the drive. It was one of those perfectly ordinary moments you don't even think to appreciate until it's gone. Out of nowhere, something went wrong with my eyes. My vision started playing strange tricks on me. At first, the white lines on the road seemed to split in two, like a bad 3D movie. I blinked hard, thinking my eyes were just tired. But it didn't go away. Everything doubled, two sets of cars, two lanes, and two of everything.

Then the world became blurry, as if I was looking through a steamed-up window. I was starting to panic as my heart started pounding out of my chest. I gripped the steering wheel tightly, repeating to myself, "Stay calm, it'll pass. Just breathe." But it didn't pass. I have no idea how I managed to drive the rest of the way, how I got my car into a parking spot without hitting anything. I stumbled into the store, my legs feeling shaky, the familiar aisles of Home Depot now a disorienting, blurry maze. I just needed to find someone, to say the words out loud to make it real. My supervisor took one look at my face and knew something was seriously wrong. She sat me down, her voice calm but firm. "You are not driving home," she said. "I will call someone for you."

My hands were trembling as I fumbled with my phone. After a few frantic, unanswered calls that made me panic even more, I finally got a hold of Robyn, my best friend since elementary school. Just hearing her voice alone brought instant comfort and made me want to burst into tears. Her reassuring voice was like a lifeline. She didn't ask a million questions. She just said, "I'm on my way," and within minutes, she arrived, dropping everything to come to my rescue. She took me away to my boyfriend's home, her comforting presence easing some of my anxiety.

The next morning, I managed an emergency appointment with my doctor, who sent me for a laundry list of blood tests, referrals to specialists. Everything moved quickly, each step heightening my anxiety. Visits to the neurologist and ophthalmologist became a dizzying routine of uncertainty.

My life became a series of waiting rooms, cold machines, and strangers asking me to follow their fingers with my eyes. Each test came back with no answers, which was somehow more terrifying than a bad result. I started to think the worst. *Am I having a stroke? Do I have a brain tumor?* The thoughts would spiral, keeping me up at night. It felt like something alien had invaded my body, something I couldn't see or fight. A new, terrifying thought started to creep in: *Am I going crazy?*

My whole life felt like it had been flipped upside down overnight. And the symptoms didn't stop with the blurry vision. A deep fatigue settled in, a tiredness so profound that no amount of sleep could touch it. I'd wake up feeling more exhausted than when I went to bed. Then came the weird tingling in my hands, a pins-and-needles sensation that would come and go without warning. My body, my reliable partner, had become a stranger, and I was scared of it.

The question "Why me?" started to play on a loop in my head. "What did I do wrong to deserve this?" I felt like I was being punished for something, but I didn't know what. The energetic, happy-go-lucky Daneshia was disappearing, replaced by a woman who was scared, confused, and constantly on edge with fear.

These mysterious episodes disrupted every facet of my life. As a full-time student balancing classes with my responsibilities at work, an aspiring actress, and a vibrant young woman enjoying her twenties, I was accustomed to juggling a full and exciting life. But now, random episodes of blurred vision, the left side of my body numb for three weeks, dizziness, chronic insomnia and fatigue dominated my existence. My previously energetic and adventurous life suddenly felt unstable, unpredictable, and fragile.

Before all of this began, my life was full and fulfilling. I was an active young woman, enjoying promotional modeling, dating, thriving at my job at Home Depot, and cross-country driving from state to state driving back repossession limousine. I had even treated myself to a red sports car, a tangible symbol of my achievements and independence. I was living my best life, or so I thought.

Yet in an instant, everything changed. These unexplained symptoms were not just inconveniences—they were intrusions into my once-perfect life. They drained me physically and emotionally, knocking me off balance literally and figuratively. Each unexpected episode made me feel increasingly helpless, deepening my frustration and sense of isolation.

Everything I had worked so hard for—my education, my career, my aspirations—suddenly seemed vulnerable and uncertain.

Months passed, filled with medical appointments, CAT scans, MRIs, and endless doctor visits. Each new test brought another wave of anxiety and another round of sleepless nights. Three years of my life were being slowly stolen by an invisible enemy. Finally, after what felt like an eternity, the doctors had an answer. I can still picture the neurologist's office and the doctor's face with his serious but kind eyes. He chose his words carefully, but they still landed like a punch to the gut.

"Daneshia," he said, "you have Multiple Sclerosis."

MS. The two letters hung in the air, heavy and final. Suddenly, everything made a horrible kind of sense. The double vision, blurriness, the fatigue, the tingling. It had a name. A name that sounded like a death sentence. The "Why me?" in my head was no longer a question; it was a scream. *What does this mean for my life? Will I end up in a wheelchair? Will I be able to have kids? Who is ever going to want to marry me?*

In the midst of despair, I found strength I never knew I possessed. I learned humility and grace, discovering that true courage meant asking for help and leaning on those who loved me. Family and friends became my anchors, their unwavering support lifting me from my darkest moments.

The emotional toll was heavy, and I grieved deeply for the life I once had. But through all the turmoil, I realized something vital: my illness was not my identity. It was a part of my journey, but not the entirety of who I was. Accepting my diagnosis was not a passive resignation but an active choice to reclaim my life. With each day, I learned more about managing symptoms, advocating for myself, and maintaining hope even in uncertainty. I embraced new routines, prioritizing self-care and health in ways I never had before.

In the process, my relationships deepened. My sisters, Renny and April, stood firmly by my side, offering unwavering support. Robyn's loyalty and Sherri's introduction to MS walks in my hometown helped me realize I wasn't alone. Each friendship fortified my strength, reminding me that vulnerability could coexist with resilience.

In the middle of all that chaos and fear, a tiny spark ignited inside me. It wasn't hope, not yet. It was something stubborn, something deep down that refused to be extinguished. It was faith. I realized, in that moment, that the answers I needed weren't going to come from a doctor or a textbook. The real test wasn't the diagnosis; it was what I was going to do with it. Prayer, meditation, and mindfulness became my essential tools, helping me to maintain my emotional balance and physical health.

So, I made a choice. I decided to fight. I didn't know what that meant yet, or how to do it. I just knew I couldn't let this disease be the end of my story. I knew I had to learn to live with this new, unwelcome reality. I had to learn to ask for help, to lean on the people who loved me. I had to accept that my life had changed forever, but that I could still have a good life.

This was just the beginning of a long, hard road. A battle that most people wouldn't be able to see. A silent battle. But it was my battle to fight, and I was, with every scared, shaking part of me, ready to start.

Looking back, I realized my journey had only just begun. This initial strike, this life-altering diagnosis, was not the end but the start of a profound transformation. And though the path ahead remained unclear, I was ready. Armed with faith, courage, and an unbreakable spirit, I knew that no matter what lay ahead, I was strong enough to face it.

Your Silent Battle Reflections:

1. Have you ever had a moment in your life where everything changed in an instant? How did it make you feel?

2. How do you usually react when your body or mind feels out of your control?

3. What helps you cope when life throws you something unexpected and frightening?

4. In moments of crisis, who or what do you lean on for support?

5. Looking back on your own struggles, what do you wish someone had said to you in your "out of nowhere" moment?

Chapter 2

THE BATTLE CRY —
WHY ME?

H ere I am at 26 years old and these are supposed to be my best years as a young adult. This is where I enjoy the aftermath of my college life, date date date to learn what type of man I want to settle with. This is where I start to walk into my career path. All of that was shattered after hearing the devastating words that I am diagnosed with MS. The only good thing about this news was having more clarity about my symptoms. All of this took me by surprise and led to me falling into a slight depression. M.S. is a rare disease. I have never felt so alone in my life. There's not one to turn to, no one that I am aware of who battled with this disease. I had no one to turn to. At that time, I thought that it was a Caucasian disease, in which this disease was mainly among people of a Caucasian descent. No one to confide in. No one in my family had this disease. So I felt like a unicorn. I thought it was rare for someone my age to have this disease.

All I could do was isolate myself so I could figure out my life. I didn't know how to make sense of my feelings, my thoughts, my emotions, much less have conversations with my loved ones about it. I just couldn't put it into words that would make sense and not be alarming. Imagine being in your twenties and having to go out on disability. I was always so happy, outgoing, and very healthy. I can count on one hand to this day how many times I've thrown up or even had a common cold. I rarely got sick. So to be diagnosed with M.S. was a news flash that I still couldn't comprehend. I didn't want to freak people out. I felt like everyone in my immediate family and close friends would look at me as a charity case and as if I was living my last days. It was as if they already started looking at me like a death sentence. I felt worse than a unicorn, I felt like a weirdo. I felt like I wanted to just run in a hole and never come out. I didn't even care anymore about my appearance. I always loved to dress and express myself through my fashion. I was always "best dressed." I was a label queen. My hair had to be laid at all times. The fragrances I wore had to be top-notch. My feminine appearance meant everything to me. I even started modeling in my early twenties. In the drop of a dime, all of this changed for me. I lost all motivation. I just wanted to be left alone. I didn't care about my appearance anymore. I could care less whether my hair was done and all I wore was basic rags/clothing to hide my shame. I no longer had a passion for fashion.

I didn't seek support from my family, friends, or support groups because I was prideful. I was always the strong one in my family and among my friends. I was the one that everyone would run to about their problems. I kept to myself because I didn't want any more pity parties. I was tired of seeing people feel hopeless or saddened for me once I shared my diagnosis with them. The last thing I wanted was for my loved ones to treat me like a handicap.

Every time I had to go on disability, which was three times, it was due to me having flare-ups with my MS symptoms. I had to stop working at Home Depot until I was cleared by my doctor to go back to work. It was normally about three months each time. To be home and not be able to work full-time was devastating. Everything in my life became part-time. Part-time worker, part-time student, part-time girlfriend. I had to drastically adjust my lifestyle to accommodate these new limitations imposed on my life by my MS diagnosis.

My new norm had to shift to part-time EVERYTHING as I stated before to accommodate my MS therapy. My new weekly schedule had to shift to me seeing my doctor once a week for my injections of Avonex 30 MCG in my upper arms for potential flare-ups. The day of my injections and the following day, I always had to make sure I had nothing planned because it made me severely fatigued. I also had to take over-the-counter pain relievers 1-2 hours before I got my injections so my flu-like symptoms wouldn't be as severe. The day after I would always wake up feeling like I was in the ring with Mike Tyson. I would feel exhausted with body aches, flu-like symptoms and sometimes nausea. I only had enough energy to turn in my sleep.

Whenever I had my injections, sometimes I had to cancel any obligations I had. My friends and loved ones would invite me to major and minor events and it was devastating letting them know I could no longer attend. Some of my friends in the beginning didn't know about my MS. So they looked at me as if I wasn't a person of my word. Some of them got mad about me canceling. I faced a lot of backlash from disappointing my family and friends. They couldn't understand why I was canceling because some, not all, knew about my illness. Sometimes I had to lie and tell them I had to work to cover up. I hated having to lie to cover up my illness. I was just afraid of being judged. They got mad at me and thought I was probably living my best life, meanwhile, I was laid up in my bed crying from the body aches, frustrations, and fatigue. I hated disappointing my loved ones. If only they knew I couldn't move.

Over time my MS treatment plan began to evolve, which was a significant breakthrough—instead of going into my doctor's office for my weekly injections, my older sister started to give me my Avonex injections at her house. It was a painful sisterly bond. She had no idea what she was doing. The nurse came to her house once, in the beginning, to coach her on how to give me my injections.

After allowing my sister to give me my injection for two years, I now have the bravery to self-inject myself for the last 16 years.

MS affects my ability to perform daily tasks and activities. My energy is always low. Every week starting Monday, I start off the week with a basket of 10 eggs and those 10 eggs represent my to-do list and task. That's all I have energy for that week. Most of the time, I can't even make it to cracking all ten of my eggs which is equivalent to 10 tasks to be checked off because my energy gets very low.

There were specific challenges and adjustments I had to make in my career due to MS. I could no longer do anything full-time. I had to transition from full-time to part-time at my job at Home Depot. Thank God I never received any stigma or discrimination in my workplace. They were very understanding. There were times I had to call out of work if I didn't feel well. I was ashamed to blame my lateness or absence on my

MS, so I used my mom having an emergency or being ill as a cover up. While attending college for a theater degree I had to transition from full-time to part-time as a student. This put a damper on my future plans because the time in school that I anticipated graduating was now pushed back to a later date. I also didn't have the energy to attend school and was very fatigued during my classes. I couldn't live college life like the usual college students. I didn't party or participate in any extracurricular activities on campus or join different student organizations like I always wanted to. I felt robbed of my college years. I couldn't enjoy my twenties like I wanted to. Those are years I can't ever get back.

My dating life while living with MS was not the same because my energy dropped tremendously. I didn't have the energy to go out as much. My romantic partners were very supportive and understanding. It was just a mental struggle for me. Just knowing that I have this illness I was always battling with myself whether they are looking at me differently even if they didn't act like it.

In the beginning stages when I first got diagnosed my initial thoughts and feelings upon receiving the diagnosis of MS were very in denial. I was afraid of the unknown and afraid of dying and being judged. I didn't want people looking at me like a handicap or a disability. I didn't want to be labeled or have this stigma. I didn't want a pity party and everyone to feel sorry for me. I went through a period of denial and disbelief about the reality of my illness that kept me stagnant. I didn't know how to rise from this label that was put on me. I didn't feel comfortable walking around with an MS bracelet on and getting a handicap sticker placed on my car because I would feel like a fraud. My MS is a silent battle because I look young, healthy and energetic. To see me jump out of a very nice car when attempting to park in a handicap parking spot. I felt they would definitely judge me or confront me to tell me that I don't deserve to park there.

I eventually came to accept and cope with the diagnosis through prayer and doing more research about it. I constantly had to reprogram my mind that "I have MS, MS doesn't have me." I had to thank God because my symptoms and outcome could be way worse. Whenever I would go to my MS walks and seminars, I would see other MS survivors who had it way worse with their symptoms and outcome. My faith was activated like never before. I had to lean on, not only to my own understanding, but God for peace and comfort despite my feeling of defeat at times. I still stood on my faith. Outside of my prayers, some coping mechanisms I used to process my emotions and come to terms with my MS was meditation through music and controlling my stress levels by avoiding any drama and stress.

The advice I would give to others who may be struggling to accept their own diagnosis of MS is to first know that you're not alone. Also tap into the countless resources that are out there in your local community or online. There are many support groups who meet in person or online where you'll feel supported. Also, attend the MS walks and seminars. I know that you can also apply for the Family and Medical Leave Act (FMLA), where you cannot get fired if you need to call out of work due to your MS flare-ups. There are many government assistance programs who give grants, and discounts for MS patients. Overall, your attitude determines your altitude. Try to be positive and have control over your mind.

Just when I already felt like crap and down in the dumps. One day I received a phone call while I was at work that a loan that I had taken out for a family member & co-signed for has not been getting paid down for several months!!!

Once I found out how much it was to pay off and how much I would have to pay every month on top of my own personal debt and car payment. Bankruptcy was my only option!!!

I asked my parents if they could potentially help me out & they told me that their hands were full at the present time. They really felt bad that they couldn't help me out. Honestly, I didn't deserve to be stressed out about someone else's debt, but this was one of the biggest lessons learned for me at an early stage of my life.

Due to my MS, I couldn't work 2-3 jobs to pay off this enormous debt. I could barely do one job full time. MS impacted my ability to manage huge expenses and debts.

By me filing bankruptcy it was very challenging and emotionally draining. I thought the world would look at me like I was a failure and irresponsible. I knew going forward I wouldn't be this lenient with my credit ever again.

How did you navigate the process of healing and moving forward after such a significant loss?
Looking back, what lessons did you learn from this experience, and how did it shape your perspective on relationships and resilience?

My boyfriend at that time was in college. He didn't really have too much to offer financially, but he was my first & I loved him.

Prior to me getting sick we had broken up a few times and got back together. I don't think we were on bad terms, but we did have one or two break ups before I got the big news!!!

I remember clearly the day I was driving from either the doctor's office or somewhere and he said to me, "Who would want a sick girlfriend?" I knew it was out of anger since we were arguing, but that definitely stung me and made me realize that it can be some truth to his statement.

It wasn't because of my element that made us eventually break up for good, but it was the worst time since I went through two other life changing events around the same time.

This breakup impacted my emotional well-being and mental health because it's the last thing I needed in addition to my MS.

I always had a strong support system in place which helped me cope with the aftermath of my breakup. They would cheer me on in trying to convince me that there's more to come. He's a dime a dozen.

Your Silent Battle Reflections:

1. When have you found yourself asking, "Why me?" in your own life? What triggered that feeling?

2. Do you believe challenges happen *to* you or *for* you? Why?

3. How do you balance moments of self-pity or frustration with hope and resilience?

4. What role does faith, spirituality, or belief play when you're searching for meaning in your struggles?

5. If you could speak to the version of yourself who first asked, "Why me?" What comfort, encouragement, or truth would you give him or her now?

Your past may shape you,
but it does not define you.
You are becoming
someone greater.

AFFIRMATION WALL

☑ I am resilient

☑ I am worthy of new beginnings.

☑ I am no longer bound by my past

☑ I walk in freedom and confidence.

☑ My story matters, and my voice has power.

☑ I am becoming the best version of me.

Pause. Breathe. Repeat these truths until they feel like your own.

Chapter 3

NAVIGATING MS + GRIEF

I grew up in a close-knit family. I have two sisters and one brother, and I am the youngest of four children. I always saw myself as "daddy's little girl."

My dad was my world, my rock, the one I turned to for guidance and support.

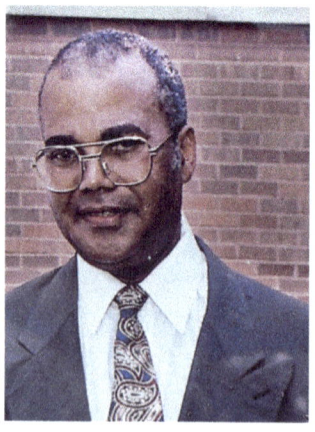

But as life would have it, just as I was still wrestling with my own MS diagnosis, my dad was battling his own health issues – glaucoma and diabetes. It was during these trying times that our bond deepened, as we found comfort and relief in confiding in each other. I just saw it as two souls navigating the storms of life together, trauma bonding through our elements.

Growing up, my dad and I shared countless special moments. He would confide in me about major financial decisions and plans, treating me not just as his daughter, but as a trusted confidante. But among these moments of closeness, there was still a dark shadow hanging over us—my dad's struggle with his alcohol addiction.

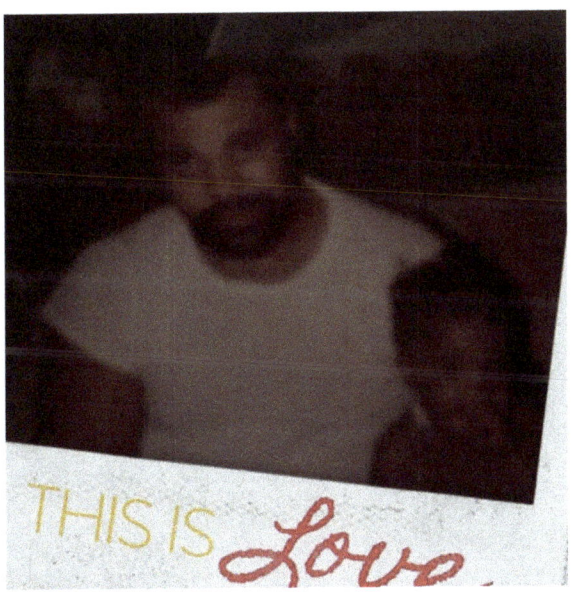

My dad's drinking wasn't just a habit; it was a coping mechanism, a means of numbing the pain and escaping his reality. Whatever that may have been. He never wanted to stress us out or be a burden, so he kept a lot of things bottled up on the inside. As his health declined, the doctors warned him time and time again to stop drinking, but the grip and his comfort with his addiction were too strong. I watched helplessly as he wrestled his demons with alcohol addiction, robbing me of the man I idolized whenever he was sober.

Whenever my dad got drunk and acted out, it really scared me because I cared about him so much. His drinking didn't just make me upset; it broke my heart, especially because I thought it was making his illnesses worse. He was sneaky about it, hiding his bottles in random places throughout the house. And he hardly ever drank in front of us, which made it even harder to deal with. But despite all that, I still had this special connection with my dad. He still remained my hero. When my dad wasn't drinking, he was the best guy ever, and I looked up to him so much. In my eyes, he could do no wrong.

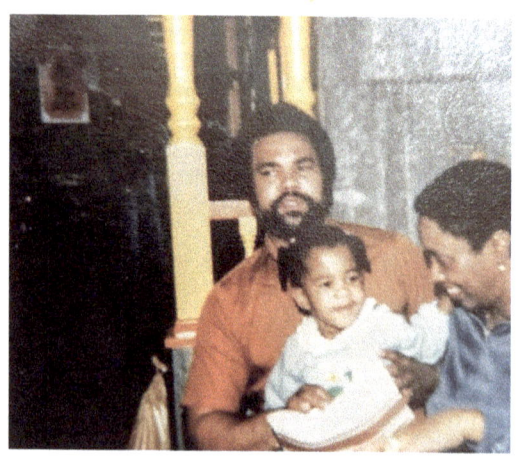

When my dad's health took a turn for the worst and he landed in the hospital, it marked the beginning of the end. When my dad was admitted to the hospital, he only had two more weeks left before he passed away. It all started one afternoon while he was sitting in the bathroom at our second home in North Carolina. He suddenly cried out, yelling, "I need help!" My older sister was there with him at the time. She called 911 and the ambulance rushed him to the hospital, where we received the devastating news that he was tremendously shaking as a lot of his main body organs were shutting down. Despite the doctors' efforts, everything was getting worse. They worked tirelessly to keep his body organs from shutting down and decided to keep him under their care. However, his condition continued to deteriorate, and he ended up on life support. It was heartbreaking to see him like that because I remember his body swelling and turning black and blue as he became more fragile.

When he was rushed to the hospital, the rest of my immediate family and I flew from New Jersey to North Carolina and stayed by his side the entire time. It was a disturbing experience and felt like a nightmare I couldn't wake up from. Eventually, I found myself facing the toughest decision of all—whether to let him go. He was being kept alive by machines, and it was clear that there was no hope for his recovery. It was a heartbreaking realization to come to terms with, especially with my mom remaining hopeful and in denial about the severity of his condition. Despite her resistance, I knew it was time to make the call. So, when the doctors asked again about pulling the plug, I made the painful decision to go ahead with it. It was one of the first hardest things I've ever had to do, but I knew it was what my dad would have wanted.

I remember it like it was yesterday, the moment they pulled the plug as my father passed from septic shock. I instantly grew numb, like I was in a daze, overwhelmed by a whirlwind of emotions. I was the one who gave the doctor the final okay to take my dad off life support. Could you imagine how I felt, being responsible for my dad taking his last breath? At that moment everything in me went numb. I couldn't even cry if I wanted to.

I pushed my emotions to the side because I wanted to stay strong for everyone else. It was as if I couldn't even process what was happening. I struggled to shed tears, to truly comprehend my new reality that he was gone, and I would never get to hold him or talk to him again. But then, in a moment of raw vulnerability, it all hit me at once.

At the funeral, as I gazed at my dad's lifeless body lying in the casket, reality hit me like a ton of bricks. Seeing him there, so still and silent, it finally sank in that he was gone and gone for good. It was like a wave of grief washed over me all at once. I couldn't move, couldn't speak – I was frozen in disbelief in front of his casket. And then, the floodgates opened, and I wept uncontrollably like a baby. It was the first step in a long journey of mourning the loss of my dad. Mourning his loss while still dealing with the symptoms of my MS felt like my health was pushed to my limits. I felt lifeless.

After my dad was buried, I had to keep myself busy to escape my pain and my reality. But no matter how busy I kept myself, the grief lingered, intensifying my MS flare-ups, and throwing me into a dark pit of depression. Stress, as I learned, is one of the top triggers for flare-ups, so I knew I had to find ways to cope, even if it meant suppressing my emotions. I threw myself into driving cross country from state to state because I love to drive. Also I took on the role of being my mother's caregiver, driving her to appointments and offering her my support. Her resilience and strength is what kept me strong, leaving me with no other choice but to keep pushing forward. Despite her own grief, she never allowed herself to break down in front of me, and I was determined to follow her example and remain strong for both of us.

However, no matter how busy I kept myself, that feeling of sadness stuck around like an uninvited guest who just wouldn't leave. It was like this heavy weight on my chest, making it hard to breathe and harder to smile. On top of all of that, my MS symptoms seemed to have gotten worse, which just made everything in my life feel like a hot mess. It got to the point where I started questioning everything – my worth, my purpose, and even my future.

I used to be full of energy, always ready to tackle whatever life threw my way. But after my dad passed away and while still struggling with my MS diagnosis and symptoms, it was like all my energy just disappeared, leaving me feeling drained and leveled off. Even getting out of bed in the morning felt like a huge struggle, like I was carrying the weight of the world on my shoulders.

I've always been a pretty upbeat person, but after my dad passed away, it was like I couldn't shake this feeling of sadness that just hung over me like a dark cloud and my mood would just tank unexpectedly. It was like no matter how hard I tried to distract myself, that feeling of emptiness just wouldn't go away.

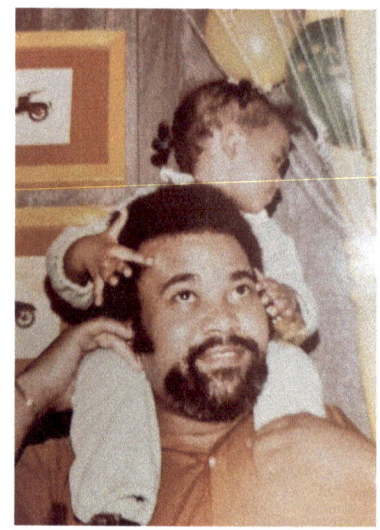

But you know what? I didn't give up. Even when it felt like the whole world was crashing down around me, I kept going. I leaned on my family and friends for support, even when I didn't want to admit that I needed it. Slowly but surely, things started to get better. I had to learn to take things one day at a time and to appreciate the little moments of joy and laughter that came my way. Most importantly, I had to learn to be kinder to myself and to give myself the space and grace I needed to heal in my own time.

I've come to understand that in life, there are only two certainties: death and taxes. It's a harsh reality, but it's one that I've had to come to terms with. While I wish I could have had more time with my dad, I've learned to cherish the memories we did share. Losing my dad was a wake-up call for me. It reminded me that tomorrow isn't guaranteed, so I've learned to appreciate each day that I'm given. Life is short, and it could always be worse. I've seen others with MS facing even greater challenges than me, which puts things into a better perspective for me. Despite the pain of losing my dad, I'm grateful for the life I have. His passing has given me a newfound sense of hope and optimism. It's taught me to be resilient and tap into a strength I didn't know I had within me.

So if you're going through something tough right now, just know that you're not alone. It might feel like the end of the world, but I promise you, it's not. You're stronger than you think, and you will get through this. Just take it one step at a time, and remember to be kind to yourself along the way.

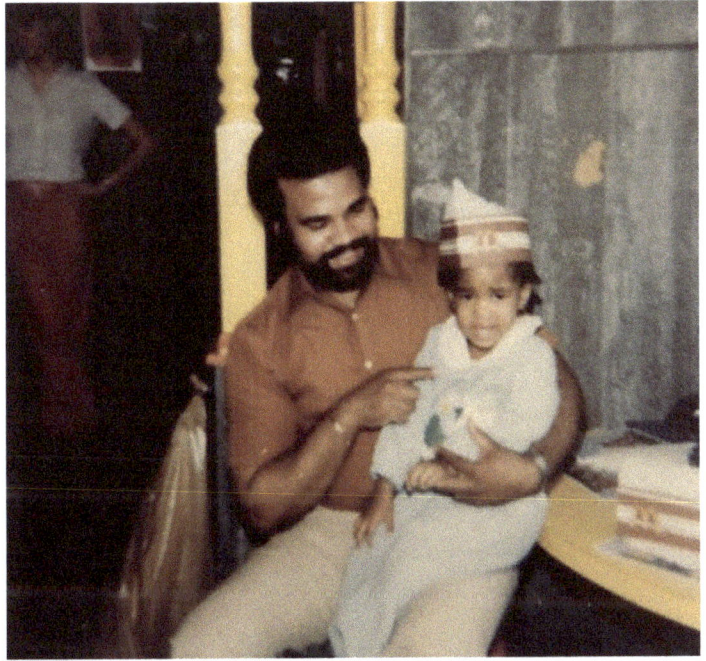

During these times of darkness, holding onto the precious memories I shared with my dad became my happy place, a gentle reminder to embrace each day like it was my last regardless of its ups and downs. It's important to really soak up those moments with the people I love the most. As we all know, life is very unpredictable, and you never know when you might not get another chance to say "I love you." My dad passing away really drove that point home for me.

Also, understand firsthand the necessity of prioritizing self-care and mental health. Grieving the loss of a loved one while managing the symptoms of a chronic illness is a difficult journey, one that demands healthy coping mechanisms and self-compassion. Whether through therapy, mindfulness, or engaging in activities that bring you joy, catering to your mental and emotional health is a priority for healing and resilience.

Your Silent Battle Reflections:

1. How have you experienced grief—not just from losing loved ones, but from losing parts of yourself, your health, or your dreams?

2. What coping mechanisms have helped you navigate seasons of grief or change?

3. How do you honor both the pain of what you've lost and the hope of what still lies ahead?

4. Who or what has been your anchor during your heaviest moments of grief?

5. In what ways has grief reshaped your perspective on life, love, and resilience?

Chapter 4

THE UNTHINKABLE

I still remember that moment vividly—the sterile white walls, the cold examination table beneath me, the paper crinkling loudly every time I moved nervously. My heart was racing because I knew that what I was about to hear could change my entire life.

The doctor spoke gently but firmly, choosing her words carefully as she explained the risks: "Daneshia, I'm not saying you can't have children, but I don't recommend it. Your MS is stable now, and pregnancy could change that drastically. I've seen it happen. One of my family members has MS, and after her baby was born, she woke up one day unable to walk or even care for her child. Her health declined rapidly."

Hearing this, my heart sank. Fear crept into every corner of my mind. Images flashed before me—of my body giving up, of losing independence, of not being able to care for a child. I was healthy, energetic, and had managed my MS so well for nearly twenty years. But suddenly, it felt like all of that didn't matter anymore.

This wasn't news any woman ever wanted to hear, even someone like me who had never been entirely sure about having kids. Truthfully, motherhood hadn't always been at the top of my list. Before my diagnosis, I was building dreams around acting, modeling, and becoming the next big star. My future felt limitless. But now, as the doctor continued explaining the risks, I felt trapped in a corner.

I thought about Teddy—my husband at the time, a man who dreamed deeply of becoming a father. He was five years older than me, a type 1 diabetic managing his own health struggles. When the doctor learned this, her eyebrows raised, her voice becoming more concerned: "Daneshia, have you two considered adoption instead? With your MS and Teddy's diabetes, having a baby could put both of you at serious risk."

Adoption? My heart resisted the idea immediately. It wasn't that adoption wasn't beautiful or meaningful—it just wasn't what I envisioned for myself. Then Teddy's mother brought up the idea of us looking into a surrogate. Another option suggesting we could still have our dream without putting my health at risk. Her heart was in the right place, but my pride and faith kicked in instantly. I found myself declaring, "Absolutely not. I got this. God's got me. I know I can do this."

Deep inside, I was terrified, but my stubbornness and determination were stronger. I was offended, almost insulted, by the suggestion that I wasn't strong enough. All my life, I had been strong, independent, and capable of overcoming every challenge. Now, I felt like I needed to prove it, not just to everyone else, but to myself.

But beneath my fierce exterior, doubt lingered. I knew that choosing motherhood would require me to step away from my medication, risking everything I had carefully built—my career, my dreams, my independence. Would this choice mean giving up acting? Would I ever be able to return to the passion that had driven me since I was a young girl? Acting had become my escape, my dream; losing it felt like losing a part of myself.

There were countless sleepless nights as I struggled with these thoughts. The question "Why me?" was always there, whispered in moments of darkness, louder than ever. Was I being punished? Was I destined never to truly experience motherhood, something that seemed so natural and effortless for other women?

I felt trapped between two worlds—my dreams of acting and Teddy's dream of having a child. The doctor's advice wasn't just medical—it felt personal. I questioned my womanhood, feeling somehow incomplete because something so fundamental was suddenly not recommended. Although I had never been someone who thought I couldn't survive without a child, now being told I probably shouldn't, stung my heart deeply.

I grieved many things in that period, but most of all, I grieved the limitations now placed upon my body. The fatigue from MS was relentless, draining my strength and leaving me feeling helpless at times. Chronic insomnia became my unwelcome companion. Sleep was elusive, and even when it came, it was fleeting. It was a daily battle, one that medication couldn't entirely fix.

Yet through it all, my family and friends kept me anchored. My sisters, April and Renny, were constant pillars of support. Renny would help me with my injections when I couldn't do them myself, and April always encouraged me, reminding me of my strength and to keep my faith. Robyn dove into researching MS just to understand my struggles better. Sherri introduced me to MS Walks, helping me see I wasn't alone. Nikki started caring for an elderly woman who suffered from MS as well to know how to care for me if my condition ever got worse. Staci always says, "You got this Nesh." Ronnette constantly reminds me of how blessed I am since she works at a hospital and witnesses so many MS patients that are not living as well as myself. Jacinth has always cheered and pushed me to eventually walk in my truth and share my story to the world.

Despite their unwavering support, there were days I chose to carry the weight of my struggles silently. I was strong, I had always been strong, and asking for help didn't come naturally to me. But through it all, faith was my ultimate anchor. Even when I had no strength left, my belief in God never wavered. I held tightly to the belief that if God had brought me this far, He wouldn't abandon me now.

Eventually, I made the decision to move forward despite the warnings. Not because I had to prove something to the doctors, but because I needed to prove something to myself. And honestly, part of me hoped it might save my marriage, might give Teddy the joy he so desperately wanted. Maybe it would give me a new sense of purpose too.

I won't lie—this decision was scary. There was no easy path. Doctors provided me with lists of precautions and endless tests: "Make sure you're tested for this," they'd say. "Check your husband's health thoroughly," they'd remind me. The preparation felt clinical and cold, and it made me doubt myself repeatedly.

But deep down, something within me whispered to keep going, keep believing. That voice said clearly, "You can do this." I clung to those words, took a deep breath, and stepped forward in faith.

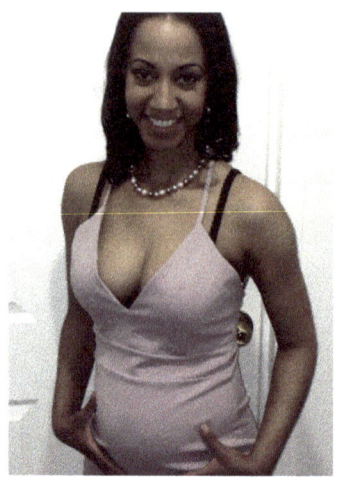

Looking back, I realize that the "unthinkable" wasn't just about pregnancy or the risk of my MS worsening. It was the courage it took to choose faith over fear. To risk losing everything for the possibility of creating a new life. To redefine my dreams, my identity, and my future.

I learned that sometimes the greatest battles we face aren't visible to the outside world. They're silent, internal struggles that shape us in ways we never imagined. In confronting the unthinkable, I found a strength I never knew I had.

Yes, MS changed me. It reshaped my dreams and forced me to face truths I wasn't prepared for. But it also taught me the value of life, the importance of faith, and the incredible strength we have when we choose to believe in ourselves—even when the world tells us otherwise.

And ultimately, this chapter of my story became a testament—not just to my own resilience, but to the power of faith, love, and the courage to step into the unknown, believing wholeheartedly that somehow, I would make it through.

Your Silent Battle Reflections:

1. How do you process being told "no" by doctors, especially when it touches something as personal as having children or pursuing your dreams?

2. Have you ever had to grieve a dream before it even had the chance to come alive? How did that feel?

3. What role does faith, hope, or resilience play when the "unthinkable" becomes your reality?

4. In moments when your plans collapse, how do you find new purpose or redefine your path?

5. What does it mean to you to hold on to possibility, even when the experts say it's impossible?

Chapter 5

LOVE & LEAP OF FAITH

After years of navigating the dating scene, where, as my friends loved to remind me, I'd "dated everything under the sun except for an astronaut and a pilot," I was a professional. White collar, blue collar, you name it. But my friends, particularly Sherri and Carlos, had a theory: "Daneshia, you're letting all the men pick you. You need to pick your Prince Charming. Come off your high pink horse and pick *your* husband."

My initial reaction? "I don't need to date online. Do you know who I am?" The idea felt beneath me. But my friends Sherri and Carlos persisted, even offering to pay for my first few months on eHarmony. The rest of our crew, mostly married or settled, were eager to live vicariously through my dating escapades. So, I relented. After a few encounters with "wacko jackals," I was ready to quit, but with nothing better to do, I kept scrolling.

Then, one night, I saw him. Teddy. His profile was a mosaic of adventure: bungee jumping, painting, camping. "Wow, he's well-rounded," I thought. "What can't he do?" His professional photos, suit and tie, screamed corporate America. "He's official," I mused. And handsome, with those hazel eyes, that bald head. Something stirred.

My father was gone by then, but my mom was healthy, and my sister was visiting. "I want y'all to look at this picture," I announced. "This picture is speaking to me." Mom, always wary of my "different" ways and online dating in particular ("That's dangerous, little girl!"), was skeptical. But I was insistent. "Ma, this is going to be the first man in my life I've ever hit on." She thought I was off my rocker. "Everybody told me I had to come off my high pink horse," I explained. "And I think I want to approach him."

"What's so different about him?" she asked.

"I don't know, Ma. But I feel something different. He's handsome... I don't know... something literally spoke to me. This is it."

My heart raced. I'd never pursued a man before. "How does this work?" I wondered, fumbling through the eHarmony interface. Mom, eventually, along with my sister, co-signed. "Yes, Daneshia, I see what you're saying. Go for it."

So, I sent an email. Days passed. Crickets. I tried another eHarmony communication channel, maybe a text or call through their anonymous number system. Still nothing.

"Damn it!" I fumed with my friends. "Y'all told me to do this, and the first man I ever hit on doesn't respond!"

Finally, he replied. His explanation? My profile was too sparse. A few modeling pictures, no real information. He thought I was a catfish or just playing around. "But," he admitted, "the only reason I responded back is because this chick is very confident and persistent. She's not telling me anything, but she wants my attention."

We exchanged real numbers. Our first date was at Dave & Buster's in New York, too loud to really talk, so he suggested Carmine's for Italian. A fancy choice for a first date, I thought. He kept looking at me. "Wow, you look so much better in person." My professional modeling shots were hot, I thought, so I gave him a look. "No, no, no disrespect," he quickly clarified. "Those pictures didn't do you justice. You're naturally pretty. I love this." That honesty, that directness, disarmed me.

The conversation flowed. I told him about my past, my ambitions. When I mentioned always dating men who were "going to come up," he cut through it. "Stop making excuses for those lame bums. I'm going to show you. We're going to go on vacation, do a lot of things." His confidence was a magnet.

After dinner, I needed the restroom but dreaded the thought of a public train station bathroom. "New York is a cesspool," I declared. Teddy, ever the problem-solver, offered a solution. "My office is two blocks away. It's open 24/7, and I have my own clean bathroom." My mind raced – going to a stranger's office? But I really had to go. I texted my friends my location, just in case. His office was impressive, his name on the door. Professional. Legit. I used his pristine bathroom, washed my hands, and then, for some reason I can't recall, felt the need to wash them again right after. He later told me he thought I was a "crazy, cool, weirdo" but found my germaphobia "cute." He walked me to the train, paid for my fare, and texted to make sure I got home safe.

The connection was undeniable. Unlike other guys, he didn't blow up my phone, which, oddly, I liked. He was busy as a financial advisor in corporate America, working 10-hour days, networking with colleagues. I learned to navigate his schedule. Then came the revelations that deepened our bond in an unexpected way. He had type 1 diabetes. When I eventually shared my MS diagnosis, it was almost a relief. "Holy shit," I thought, "he's just as fucked up as I am, or even more." It sounds crazy, but knowing he had his own chronic illness, his own daily battles, made me feel an incredible sense of comfort and empathy. He would understand.

He was also financially successful, doing extremely well on top of yearly bonuses. No kids, didn't seem like a player, didn't smoke weed. "This is wonderful," I thought. He started inviting me to stay over more, especially since I was pursuing acting and modeling in the city. "You don't always have to rush back home," he'd say. "I have two bedrooms, a pull-out couch. We don't have to have sex." It was perfect timing, as I was considering moving to New York anyway.

There were red flags, even then. He drank more than I liked, wasn't as "masculine" in some traditional ways (like driving) because he was a city boy. Our early sexual encounters weren't mind-blowing because of the commute. He'd blame the infrequency of our meetings. "Once you move up here," he promised, "everything will get better. Our communication, intimacy... I won't be coming home to an empty house. I'll probably stop drinking as much."

Despite the flags, his offer was a win-win. A place to stay in the city where my career was taking off. I was ready to leave home anyways. A year or so into dating seriously, he pressed the issue: "Daneshia, I can't take someone serious that I'm only seeing once or twice a week. I need you to move up here." So, after thinking about it for several months or maybe even a year, I transferred my Home Depot job, and a week later, I moved in with Teddy. A year after that, on his 40th birthday, he proposed. Nine months later, we were married. It felt like I'd found my Prince Charming, the first man I'd ever pursued, now my husband.

Our marriage, like any, had its challenges, amplified by our respective health conditions. Teddy was always more vocal about his diabetes; I tended to internalize my MS struggles. His emotional intelligence wasn't his strong suit, and it often felt like his health took precedence. But the dream of a family, particularly his dream, began to take center stage.

The doctors had been clear: pregnancy wasn't recommended for me (as detailed in Chapter 4). The risks were significant. Yet, a fierce hope burned within me. It was a leap of faith, fueled by my own sense of strength, my willpower, and the undeniable fact that I'd been living remarkably well with MS compared to many others. I felt it in my bones: I got this. No one could tell me otherwise. There were days, especially in the early stages of my MS, when I'd almost forget I had it. I was managing so well – working, going to college, auditioning, even being a landlord.

Teddy was my biggest cheerleader. He'd supported my acting dreams; how could I not support his dream of fatherhood? And practically, if I needed to stop working due to the pregnancy or MS, he was financially secure enough to support us. I wouldn't have to work another day if I couldn't. Deep down, a part of me also hoped a child might heal the cracks in our marriage, bring us closer, make him step up. The therapists had warned us a child could worsen existing problems, but I clung to optimism.

The decision to come off my MS medication was the second scariest decision that I ever had to make. If something went wrong, there was no safety net. But the desire to give Teddy his dream, coupled with my own faith and the financial security he offered, pushed me forward.

Your Silent Battle Reflections:

1. What risks or leaps of faith have you taken for love, and how did they shape your journey?

2. How do you balance medical advice or outside voices with the desires of your heart?

3. Have you ever made a sacrifice in a relationship, hoping it would strengthen the bond? What was the outcome?

4. What role does hope play when you're determined to chase something others say is impossible?

5. How can love, whether romantic or familial, serve as both a challenge and a source of strength in your life?

Chapter 6

Inner Warrior
— My Kind of
Motherhood

They said it wasn't recommended. They told me not to risk it. But God had the final say.

T3 was never part of my plan. Not really. But he was always part of God's plan. And the way he came into my life, defying all odds, breaking every medical warning, healing pieces of me I didn't know were broken, proved just that.

The doctors warned me that pregnancy could trigger severe MS flare-ups. "Although you're strong enough, and we would like to see you grow your family, we don't recommend you taking that risk by coming off your medication," they said. And I listened, I nodded, I took it seriously. But something deep inside of me—faith, love, or maybe just stubborn hope—whispered, *Try anyway.*

So we did.

At the time, my marriage was already cracked, full of arguments and silences we couldn't seem to fix. But I believed a baby might be the glue. I know now that isn't how love works, but when you're drowning, you cling to anything that looks like it might keep you afloat. My husband had always said he wanted a son, his mini-me, someone to carry his name. Since he had supported my acting dreams, I thought I would help him chase his. It felt like an act of love, sacrifice, and partnership. And maybe, deep down, I thought if I gave him his dream, he'd give me back the love I longed for.

My son, T3, wasn't just a baby; he was a prayer finally answered. My husband and I bought a ton of pregnancy tests, maybe ten, fifteen of them. Why so many? Because the second I knew, I had to stop my MS medicine. That stuff could hurt a baby, and the thought of causing him any harm, any birth defects, it twisted me up inside. So, I peed on a stick every few days, my heart thumping, a crazy mix of hope and sheer terror. We were trying, yes. He wanted this baby, dreamed of a son to carry on his name. And me? I'd agreed.

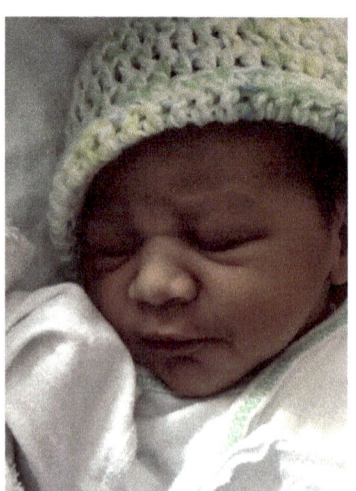

Finding out I was pregnant was a whirlwind of conflicting emotions. Ironically, Teddy and I were in the middle of a heated argument when I saw the positive test. He was sleeping in the other room, the door locked. I had to knock, to interrupt our silent war, to share the news he'd longed for. "Teddy, I need you to come look at this." The joy was there, but it was tainted by the circumstances. He was ecstatic, wanting to call everyone, while I was still processing the absurdity of the moment. "Am I making the biggest mistake of my life?" I wondered.

My pregnancy itself was beautiful, just as the doctors predicted for many MS patients—no morning sickness, no major issues, until the last two weeks. Then, I was sick as a dog, a horrible cough, exhausted beyond measure. I went into labor already depleted, coughing into a spit cup even on the delivery table. But I did it – six and a half hours of natural labor, no epidural. My sister videotaped, Teddy and my mom were there. Through the pain, the exhaustion, the confusion, I felt like Superwoman. I had defied the odds.

The first two months with T3 were a blur of sleepless nights and, unfortunately, more arguments with Teddy. He complained constantly about being tired. "How the hell are you so tired?" I'd think. "You didn't do the work!" There were moments I questioned everything, feeling a sadness that bordered on postpartum depression. T3 zapped every last ounce of my already low energy. It took about four months before I started to feel like myself again.

But then, the pure, unadulterated joy of Theodore Hatwood III—T3—began to truly shine through the fog. Holding him, seeing him, I knew I hadn't made a mistake. He was, and is, the best decision I ever made. He's made me realize I'm stronger than I ever thought. He's pushed me to prioritize, to understand how short life is, to strive for greatness not just for myself, but for him. I'm no longer the people-pleaser I once was. He's given me a deeper sense of purpose; I'm living for him.

Even on days when MS drains me, when I don't feel like getting out of bed, I look at him, and I know I have to. It's not an option. God and T3 give me a strength I didn't know I possessed. And those small moments – when he's looking at me with pure love, or when he blurts out, "Mommy, I love you," or "Mommy, you a good mommy," or "Mommy, you look pretty" – those are the affirmations that erase any doubt. In those moments, I know I'm not a douchebag mom; I'm just a mom, doing her best, fueled by a love and a miracle I almost didn't dare to dream of.

Why go against doctors, against common sense? Because my husband's biggest dream was a family, a son. As his wife, I felt I owed him that. Did I always dream of being a mom? Honestly, no. It just wasn't my thing. Especially after my diagnosis. But as I got older, became a godmother to two amazing kids, and people started saying, "Daneshia, you'd be a great mom." Teddy said it too. So, I looked at him, knew he'd be a good dad, and something in me just said, "Okay. I have MS, but MS doesn't have me. Let's try."

But here's the raw truth: there was a bitter taste to it all, even from the start. If I'd been with a man who wasn't so set on having a kid, I probably wouldn't have. Our marriage was already rocky, full of arguments and silences long before we even talked about a baby. I guess a part of me, the part that still believed in fairy tales, thought this huge sacrifice – risking my health, the sleepless nights, the worry – would somehow fix us. That if he saw what I was willing to do for him, for our family, he'd... I don't know... change. Love me better.

Life doesn't work like that, does it? We fought, even when I was pregnant. Stupid fights that left me feeling small and unloved, like everything I was putting my body through didn't even matter to him. I kept hoping, praying, that once T3 was here, once he held his son, *his* Theodore III, things would click. That our marriage would get stronger.

Instead, within a year of T3's birth, it started falling apart, faster and harder than I could have imagined. It left me gasping.

Let me be absolutely clear: T3 is the best thing that ever happened to me. Not for a second do I regret him. But no woman who's almost 38, who's lived with MS for twelve years, walks into pregnancy with a marriage already on life support without hoping for a miracle. And when that miracle doesn't show up for your marriage, it hurts. There were nights, those first few months with T3, when I'd lock myself in the bathroom, the sound of my own sobs muffled by the running water, thinking, "I've made the biggest mistake of my life thinking I can manage being a wife and a mother while battling MS."

His birth itself was a battle against the odds. We weren't supposed to conceive that easily, due to our health issues we both were battling. But we did. Quickly. Like it was meant to happen. Like God said, "Let me show you what I can do for you." Getting pregnant felt like a long shot. But two months after we started trying, there it was, that second pink line. I was pregnant! When that positive test finally came, I froze. Not in fear, but in awe. It was so fast, it felt like a sign. This baby wanted to be here. He fought his way through the doctors' warnings, through our messy marriage, even through my own acting career, which was finally taking off in New York. I knew a baby would change all of that, but I told myself, "He supported my dreams before; he'll support them even more now that I've given him his son." Another dream that turned to dust.

The birth itself? Six hours of raw, unmedicated pain. No epidural. I didn't even go to the hospital until I was six centimeters dilated, just breathing and praying through contractions that felt like my body was splitting in two. My sister was there, filming, God bless her. The nurses kept saying they'd never seen anyone so calm in so much pain. I wasn't screaming, just riding the

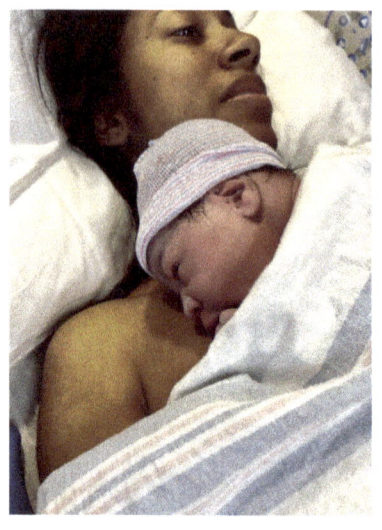

waves. And to top it off, two weeks before, I'd had this horrible whooping cough. Couldn't sleep, just hacking my lungs out. My mom had to hold a spit cup for me while I was pushing because I was still so full of mucus. But then he was here. Seven pounds of perfection. My T3. Holding him, all that pain, it just... vanished. It was well worth it.

I'd moved back to New Jersey from our place in New York about two months before he was born. All my doctors were here. Teddy came about a month later. He complained about moving to New Jersey in the beginning, but I told him, "Look, I moved to New York for you. Now it's your turn to move to New Jersey for me." My mom and sister were healthier then, and they promised to help us with the baby. Nobody knew how my MS would handle having a baby. The doctors made it sound like I could be bedridden. I needed to be home, near my family. I wanted T3 to grow up around his family.

Then the real juggling act started. New mom, MS warrior, wife in a war-torn marriage. And then, slowly, my own mom started to get sick with Parkinson's disease. The woman I counted on for support started needing my support, just as I was stretched to my breaking point. Teddy at the time had his diabetes, which had its own set of demands on me, even when I felt like an empty well. And I was still juggling working at Home Depot part time.

The biggest challenge? The fighting. Screaming, cussing, slamming doors. I know the neighbors heard. My mom would hear it, her face lined with worry, sometimes knocking on our door, begging us to stop. He'd be drinking, and when he drank, we wouldn't stop arguing, just on and on, this stream of anger.

The worst part was T3. When he was just a toddler, maybe two, he'd get between us. This tiny little boy, his face crumpled in tears, his little hands pushed out, trying to stop both of us from arguing. He'd start crying. That broke me. When your baby has to try and save you from each other, you know it's over.

I begged Teddy to just go back to his place in New York for a while. "Let's just take a breather," I'd say. "This isn't healthy for T3 or for us." "Serve me with papers if you want me out of your life," he'd say. We tried to lie, make up stories to protect T3. It was awful. Eventually, he moved into the basement. We lived like that for over a year, co-parenting from different parts of the house, him coming up for his "T3 time" then going back down. T3 got used to it, I guess.

I felt like I was giving everything to everyone. My sick husband, my new baby, my own failing body, my mother who was slowly fading, my job, the house. There was nothing left for Daneshia. I got so thin. People at work would whisper, "Are you okay, Daneshia? You look sick." I'd see myself in the mirror and barely recognize myself. I dropped to ninety-five pounds. Ninety-five. At five-foot-five, I looked like the wind could carry me away. I looked like a ghost. I wore a double zero. "Please don't lose any more weight!" friends would say. I wanted to scream, "I'm not trying to!"

I was eating, but the stress was just eating me. My MS was flaring up, numbness creeping back into my scalp. I was having trouble at work. I got hurt there, two times, not including my huge car accident in 2020 driving to work totaling out my Lexus. Each time I got hurt, it was bad enough to need time off. A customer's order fell off the shelf onto my right foot, then I sprained my tailbone when a coworker fell on me. It felt like life was just kicking me while I was down, over and over.

So many nights, I just cried. Cried to God, because He was the only one I felt was listening. *Damn this marriage. Damn this sickness. Damn, T3, I don't want you to be another statistic. I didn't get married for this.* The beautiful wedding, the expensive dress, it all felt like everything was going down the drain. *How am I going to do this alone? I can barely take care of myself.*

What got me through? My prayer. Lots of prayers and my music. Music was my escape, my church. When the house was quiet, I'd blast gospel, house music or anything with a beat that could drown out the noise in my head. I'd just drive around sometimes, windows down, letting the music fill me up. And I kept busy. Fixing up the house, building my little "she-shed" in the backyard – that was therapy too. A place just for me.

My sisters, my friends, they'd all remind me of how strong I was. "Look at everything you've done, Daneshia! You have moved to New York, built a career, and now a family, all with MS!" My aunt would shake her head, was she misdiagnosed? "I don't know how she does it, taking care of her mom when she's got so much on her own plate." They didn't know half of it, the real ugly stuff, but their words were like little sips of water in a desert. Sometimes a friend would be crying on my shoulder, then stop and say, "Wait, Daneshia, you've got all your stuff going on, and you never complain. How are you?" That meant the world. Just knowing someone saw me.

Motherhood. It's the hardest job, the toughest "hood" there is. Hashtag no snooze button, no days off, no calling in sick. It's beautiful and exhausting, all at once. T3 is my world and my heartbeat.

Being his mom, it changed everything. Sometimes he'll yell, "Mommy Mommy!" and I still get this little jolt, like, *Wow, that's me. I'm a mom.* When he's sick, when I have to rush him to the doctor, everything else fades. My MS, my tiredness, it doesn't matter. It's all about him. It forces me to be stronger than I think I am. It makes me dig deeper.

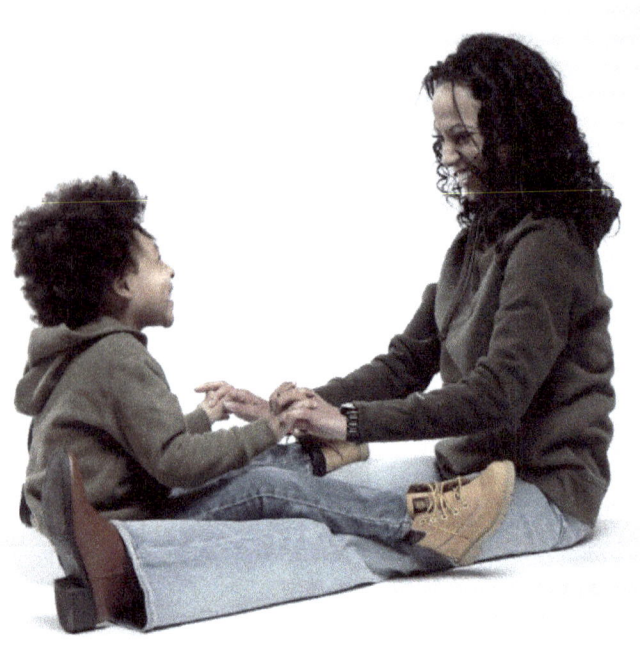

I've learned I'm tougher than I ever knew. But I've also learned I have to take care of myself. I used to run myself into the ground for everyone else, until my cup was bone dry. I can't do that anymore. If my cup is empty, I can't be good for T3, I can't be good for my mom, I can't be good for anyone. So now, I guard my "Dani time" fiercely. I'll call out of work. I'll cancel plans. I'll sit in my car alone, just to have a few moments of peace to myself. And I don't feel guilty about it anymore.

If I could tell other moms, other women juggling a million things, anything, it would be this: Be selfish sometimes. It's not a dirty word; it's survival. Listen to your body. Trust your gut. It's okay to say no. It's okay to not be okay. And it's okay to ask for help, to lean on your village. Taking care of yourself isn't selfish; it's the only way you can keep taking care of everyone else. Don't let your cup get so empty you start hating the world.

To every woman carrying the weight of a marriage, an illness, a parent, a job, and a child, please know that you are not alone. You don't have to be a superwoman every day. You don't have to wear your cape 24/7. And it's okay to say, *Today, I choose me.*

This whole journey – MS, a failed marriage, taking care of my mom, raising T3, all felt like an uphill battle at times. But it also showed me what I'm made of. T3, he was a miracle. Getting pregnant was a miracle. God trusted me with this boy, with this life. And even on the hardest days, when I feel like I can't take another step, I remember that God trusted me and appointed me for this journey. And somehow, that's enough to keep me going. This story, all of it, the good, the bad, the ugly, it needs to be told. If it helps just one other person feel less alone, then every single struggle, every tear, it means something. And I thank God every day that he trusted me to do it.

Your Silent Battle Reflections:

1. How has motherhood (or caregiving) revealed strengths you didn't know you had?

2. In what ways do you pour into others, and how do you make sure your own cup is refilled?

3. Have you ever sacrificed your well-being for your family? What did it teach you about balance?

4. What does being a "warrior" in your own life look like—especially when faced with challenges?

5. How can you honor both your role as a caregiver and your own identity outside of those responsibilities?

Chapter 7

BREAKING CHAINS

A marriage doesn't just blow up in one day. It's like getting sick. It starts with a little cough, a slight fever you try to ignore. You tell yourself, "We're just tired," or "It's just a rough patch." But when you're both already living with illnesses that don't go away, a simple cold can turn into pneumonia real fast. Before you know it, the whole thing is on life support.

If I'm being honest, our marriage was coughing before we even walked down the aisle. Looking back, I can now see how our marriage fell apart suddenly, without warning, but the truth is, the signs showed long before the wedding. Before the dress. Before the vows. Even before the beautiful engagement ring.

We both carried invisible weights, my Multiple Sclerosis and his Type 1 diabetes. Those weren't occasional storms; they were daily companions, always lurking in the background of our relationship. We woke up sick every day, just in different ways. With illnesses like ours, there's no pause button, no "get well soon." It's not the flu where you recover in a week. It's not surgery where healing is a straight line. Chronic illnesses are messy, unpredictable, and relentless. And when you bring two chronically ill people into one relationship, you quickly learn that love alone doesn't erase the fatigue, the flare-ups, the high or low blood sugars, and the sleepless nights.

When we were dating, I lived in Jersey and he lived in New York. I can still remember canceling plans at the last minute because my body simply said, "No." Fatigue would hit me like a ton of bricks, or insomnia would keep me awake all night, leaving me drained the next morning. On his side, he had his highs and lows with diabetes, blood sugars that could skyrocket or crash without warning. He would leap out of bed in the middle of the night like someone was chasing him, reaching for his insulin or ice cream to stabilize himself.

We both knew what it meant to live in survival mode. That's what bonded us in a strange way. In the beginning, it even felt comforting: *finally, someone who gets it.* Someone who understood waking up sick every day. Someone who couldn't look at me with empathy, because he was also fighting his own battles. But I've learned that comfort can also blind you. I ignored what those early struggles really meant.

By the time we got engaged, I told myself, *No one's perfect. Every relationship has issues.* I was in my thirties, tired of dating. I'd dated men of every background. From blue collar, white collar, you name it. My friends were getting married, and I didn't want to be the last one standing at the altar of loneliness. He wasn't perfect. I wasn't perfect. But the pros seemed to outweigh the cons. He had a good job, he promised to support my acting dreams, and he wanted a family. And there was that strange connection, two sick people bound by resilience. I thought it meant something special. I thought it meant we'd always have each other's backs.

So I ignored the signs, packed my bags, and said yes to everything. Yes to moving to New York. Yes to engagement. Yes to marriage. My first time ever living with a man. My first time leaving the safety net of my family. My first big leap.

I remember thinking: *The grass always looks greener on the other side. Maybe this is as good as it gets. Maybe it's time to stop searching for perfection and just build with someone who wants to build with me.* From the start, our illnesses shaped the rhythm of our marriage. The problem was, I often carried more weight.

At some point, if his blood sugar crashed, I'd wake up in the middle of the night with him, keeping him company as he gulped down juice or shoved ice cream into his mouth to stabilize. I'd sit with him when his sugars were sky-high and he had to inject insulin. I'd lose my own sleep, on top of my insomnia, just to make sure he wasn't alone in it. Eventually this became short lived.

When my body crashed, when fatigue had me pinned to the couch or my scalp went numb from a flare-up? He didn't always rise to the occasion. I thought marriage meant we'd take turns holding each other up, but it often felt one-sided because his illness required more urgent attention.

It wasn't that he was cruel or intentionally neglectful. He had his own struggles. But his struggles often drowned out mine. His illness was louder, more visible. Diabetes demanded immediate action: eat sugar now, inject insulin now. My MS was silent, invisible, harder to explain. And in that silence, I often felt unseen.

That imbalance grew heavier after the wedding. I expected empathy, romance, tenderness and affection. Instead, what I got was more arguing, more stress, and less intimacy. I told myself love required sacrifice. And when I gave birth to our son, Theodore III, our miracle baby, I felt like I had given him the ultimate gift.

But here's the part that stings the most. I thought that gift would heal our marriage. I thought it would bring us closer, make our love deeper, earn me more respect and appreciation. Instead, the opposite happened.

Within months of giving birth, the cracks widened even more. Arguments grew louder. Respect dwindled. And I, the woman who had sacrificed her body, her health, her dreams, and her energy to give him what he wanted most, felt invisible.

I remember lying in the living room on a futon with our newborn while Teddy slept alone in the bedroom, undisturbed. Night after night, I got up with the baby, changed diapers, fed him, soothed him, all while battling my own MS fatigue and recovering from a natural birth. I sacrificed my healing so he could rest, so he could function at work. I took off close to one year at my job so I could heal properly.

And yet, even after all that, he'd still complain about being tired.

Do you know what that does to your spirit? To hear constant complaints from someone who doesn't see the sacrifices you're making? It chips away at your respect. It makes love feel like a transaction where your contributions are invisible, no matter how much you pour in.

The weight of it all—motherhood, MS, a failing marriage, caregiving for my mom, keeping the house together, and working at Home Depot—dragged me down. My body showed the evidence before my mind admitted it.

I'd look in the mirror and hardly recognize the woman staring back at me. From dark circles, hollow cheeks bones, tired eyes. I was exhausted from being the "strong one" for everyone else while neglecting myself. I wasn't.

And still, I kept going. For my son. For my mom. For the house. For survival.

As the marriage unraveled, our home became a battleground. Arguments escalated until neighbors could hear us shouting through the walls. My mother, still mobile at the time, would knock on the door, pleading for us to stop.

The saddest part? Sometimes our son, barely two years old, would wedge his tiny body between us, hands outstretched like a referee, crying for us to stop. No child should ever have to play peacemaker between parents. That broke me in ways I still can't fully put into words.

At one point, he moved to a different part of the house while I stayed in our room with our son. We lived like roommates, co-parenting under one roof, pretending to hold it together for appearances. But the truth was undeniable: we were done.

In the middle of all of this, two things kept me alive: prayer and music. I prayed constantly, even when words failed. Sometimes my prayers were nothing but tears on my pillow. Other times they whispered pleas for strength just to make it through the day. Music is my therapy, my salvation. I blasted songs in the house, in the car, anywhere I could. Music drowned out the arguments, soothed my spirit, and reminded me I was still alive. Gospel songs reminded me of God's promises. R&B reminded me that I still deserved love. Even on the darkest nights, music carried me when words and people could not.

Eventually, I had to face the truth: love wasn't enough. Sacrifice wasn't enough. And hoping things would get better wasn't enough.

The therapist we saw once told us point-blank: *If you two have a baby right now, it will break this marriage.* And she was right. Within months of our son's birth, the foundation cracked beyond repair.

I tried everything: conversations, counseling, separation, writing letters pouring my heart out. But he refused to leave unless I served him papers. He stated that he knows how the court system works and he didn't want to take the chance of losing joint custody by leaving without any authorized paperwork. So, I served him. Filing for divorce wasn't what I wanted. I wanted healing, peace, respect, just temporary space. But it was the only way to break free.

Walking away from a marriage you prayed for, sacrificed for, and fought for isn't easy. It's a grief all on its own. I carried guilt, shame, and fear. Fear of raising my son alone. Fear of how people would judge me. Fear of what MS would look like without a partner by my side.

But I also carried a quiet knowing: I couldn't stay. Staying would have killed my spirit.

Breaking the chains wasn't just about ending a marriage. It was about reclaiming my self-worth, my dignity, my health, and my peace.

Looking back now, I realize the lessons were always there, even in the middle of the chaos. I just couldn't see them clearly through my pain. My first advice to anyone reading this book is to respect your red flags. They don't fade with time, and love doesn't erase them. If anything, those red flags only grow louder and brighter the longer you ignore them. I saw the signs early on, but I told myself things would get better once we moved in together, once we got engaged, once we got married, once we had his mini me. But the truth is, marriage doesn't erase impairment; it magnifies it.

Another lesson I had to learn the hard way is that sacrifice without appreciation will drain you dry. Love is not about losing yourself for someone else's dream while your own life crumbles. I risked my health, my career momentum, and pieces of myself to help build the life my husband wanted and I wanted if our marriage was healthy, but it wasn't. I was thinking my sacrifice would buy me love, more time for us to mend things back together, security, and respect. Instead, I found myself emptier than I had ever been, with nothing to show for it but resentment and exhaustion. Love should never require you to disappear to prove your worth.

I also learned that self-care isn't optional; it's survival. You can't pour from an empty cup, no matter how much you want to be everything to everyone. I kept trying to carry my marriage, my son, my mother, my job, and my illness all at once. I poured into everyone else, but I neglected myself until I was down to ninety-seven pounds, my body physically showing the toll of what my spirit had already known. I was running on empty. Now I understand that taking care of myself is not selfish. It's the only way I can show up fully for the people I love.

And perhaps one of the most freeing lessons of all is this: two good people can still be wrong for each other. Divorce doesn't mean we were both villains. It doesn't mean either of us was entirely bad. It means we were not the right fit, not the right balance, not the right partners for the journey we tried to take together. That doesn't erase the good that once existed, but it does mean that staying would have destroyed us both.

Most of all, I learned that sometimes the only way to live free is to break the chains that bind you. And those chains don't always come in the form of handcuffs or visible restraints. Sometimes they're the expectations, the patterns, the toxic cycles you settle into because you're afraid to face the unknown. But breaking free, though it nearly broke me in the process, was the only way I could step into the life I was meant to live.

Divorce was never in my plan. I didn't walk down the aisle to one day walk away. I didn't risk my body and my health to bring a child into the world only to raise him in two separate homes. None of that was part of my vision. But life doesn't bend to our plans. Life forces us to grow, to face truths we'd rather bury, to honor the quiet voice inside that says, *this is not where you're meant to stay.*

What I know now is that life isn't about clinging to what looks good on the outside. It's not about the beautiful wedding dress, the sparkling ring, or the carefully posed family pictures. It's about the truth inside, the peace or the lack of it, the love or the absence of it, the respect for it. Staying in a situation that looks good to others but slowly destroys you is not strength; it's surrendering yourself for appearances.

Walking away was not the end of me. In fact, it was the beginning. I may have walked away from a marriage, but I walked into myself. I walked into a deeper awareness of my worth, a fiercer love for myself, and a faith that carried me through storms I thought would drown me. The chain of sacrificing my truth to maintain a broken union is one I will never let bind me again.

Your Silent Battle Reflections:

1. Have you ever ignored red flags in a relationship because you wanted to believe in love or stability?

2. In what ways have you stayed in situations longer than you should have, and what finally pushed you to let go?

3. How do you define "breaking chains" in your own life—whether in relationships, health, or personal growth?

4. What role has self-worth played in your ability to walk away from something unhealthy?

5. Looking back on a painful ending, what hidden strength or lesson can you now see more clearly?

Chapter 8

THE POWER OF
CHOOSING SELF

There comes a point in life when the mirror staring back at you is no longer just about appearance, but your truth. For years, I avoided fully confronting my illness. I managed it, lived with it, even denied it at times, but I never looked it square in the face and said, *I have MS, but MS does not have me.* That shift didn't happen overnight. It came through slow realizations, small awakenings, and the growing awareness that hiding or shrinking wouldn't save me.

I remember when my medication first began to stabilize my flare-ups. The episodes became less frequent, and for the first time, I felt like I could breathe again. Around that same time, I started attending MS seminars and the annual MS walks. At first, I went quietly, hesitant to claim this part of my identity out loud. But when I got there, surrounded by people who were battling the same invisible enemy, something shifted.

I saw wheelchairs. I saw canes. I saw people whose bodies had betrayed them in ways mine hadn't yet. And then I saw their eyes, full of resilience, full of fight. When I shared my story, when I said, "I have MS, I'm on medication, I'm still working and pursuing my dreams, I went to college, I'm married and I even had a baby," people looked at me with awe. They hugged me, asked for pictures, and asked me what my secret was. In their eyes, I wasn't just surviving, but I was thriving. And that's when it hit me: I had been so focused on what MS might take away that I had failed to see all the ways I was still living abundantly.

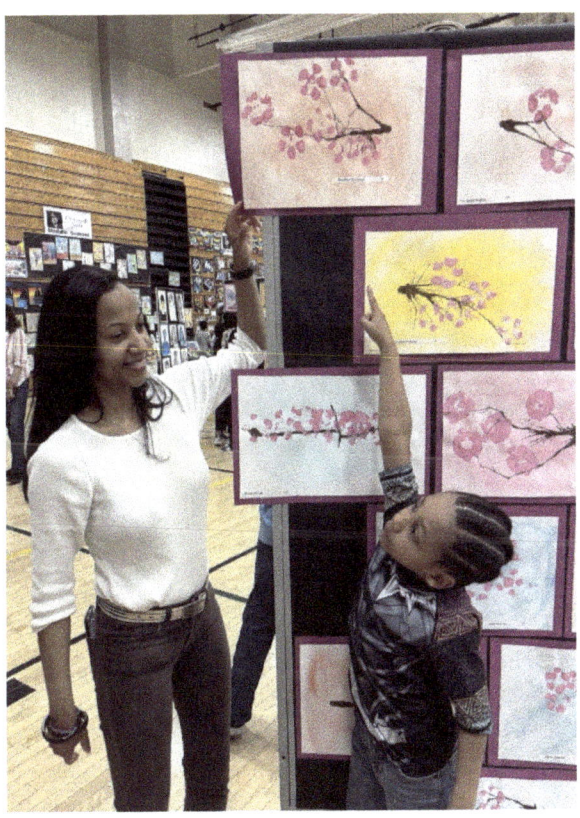

For a long time, fear held me hostage. The fear of the unknown. The fear of waking up one day unable to walk. The fear of what my dating life would look like, or if anyone could ever love me beyond the diagnosis. MS is unpredictable; you never know when your body might betray you. And for years, that uncertainty sat like a shadow over my future. But slowly, with prayer, with community, and with the determination to keep moving, I learned that fear doesn't get the final say.

The first steps to reclaiming myself were simple, but powerful. I started reminding myself daily: *I am more than my illness. I am a daughter. A mother. A sister. A friend. I am an artist, a dreamer, a woman of faith. MS is part of me, but it is not all of me.* Choosing myself meant refusing to let my diagnosis write my whole story.

That choice began to shift everything. As a wife and mother, I had often let myself get swallowed up by roles and responsibilities. I was someone's partner, someone's caretaker, someone's everything. But when the marriage crumbled, I had to redefine who I was outside of those roles. Choosing myself didn't mean I stopped being a mother; it meant I finally realized that to be the best mother, I had to pour into myself first. If my cup was empty, I couldn't pour into my son's life.

Therapy helped. Friends who spoke life into me helped. My family, reminding me that I had always been strong, helped. And music, always music, was my therapy on the days when no one else's words could reach me. Prayer anchored me, but music carried me. It gave me space to feel and heal.

There were moments when guilt tried to creep in, when saying "no" felt selfish. For years, I was a people-pleaser. I wanted to be everything for everyone. Canceling plans made me feel like I was letting people down.

Saying I needed rest felt like weakness. But eventually, I reached a point where I had no energy left to give. I had to learn that choosing myself was not neglecting others. It was the only way to keep showing up with love, instead of resentment. Now, I don't apologize for it anymore. When I say "sorry, not sorry," I mean it with my whole chest. Because if I'm not good, my son isn't good. My mother isn't good. My life falls apart.

Still, one of my deepest battles was wondering if anyone could truly love me despite my illness. That question haunted me for years. Would a man see me as too much? Too complicated? Too fragile? But over time, I realized that someone who truly loves me will love all of me, not just the pretty parts, not just the convenient parts, but the messy, unpredictable, invisible battles too. My illness doesn't make me less worthy of love. In fact, it has made me stronger, wiser, and more empathetic. Whoever cannot see that doesn't deserve me.

Faith is what helped me believe that I am deserving of unconditional love. I have always believed that what you put into the universe, you will get back. And I know I've sown some good seeds. I have loved people deeply, supported them, and shown up when it mattered. I have been a good daughter, a good wife, a good friend, a good sister and a good mother. So I believe, without a doubt, that good love, real love, will find its way back to me.

The biggest change since choosing myself is simple but life-changing: I learned how to say no. No without guilt. No without explanation. No without feeling like I have to earn the right to rest. I stopped apologizing for taking up space, for protecting my peace, for honoring my boundaries. That shift alone has transformed my life more than anything else.

If I could speak to the version of myself who once felt unseen, invisible, and forgotten, I would hold her face in my hands and tell her: *Good job. You made it. Stop second-guessing yourself. God has never left you. He never will. You are stronger than you know, braver than you believe, and more beautiful than you see in the mirror. Don't let anyone, not even yourself, convince you otherwise.*

Choosing myself didn't mean walking away from responsibilities. It meant walking into my truth. It meant realizing I deserve the best, not the bare minimum, not leftovers, not love laced with conditions, but the very best. Because at the end of the day, MS may live in my body, but it doesn't own my soul.

And when I finally embraced that truth, I stopped asking, *Will anyone love me despite my illness?* and started declaring, *I love me because of all I've overcome. And that will always be enough.*

Your Silent Battle Reflections:

1. What was a turning point in your life when you finally chose yourself over others' expectations?

2. Do you struggle with guilt when putting yourself first? How can you reframe that as an act of strength?

3. How do you remind yourself that you are more than your roles (wife, mother, caregiver, etc.)?

4. Who in your life encourages you to prioritize your healing, and how can you lean on them more?

5. What does unconditional self-love look like to you, and how can you practice it daily?

Chapter 9

BATTLE OF THE TRUTH

For most of my life, I kept my business close to my chest. I've never been the "tell-all" friend. I'm warm and personable, yes, but I hold sacred things close—faith, family, pain. When MS arrived, that instinct to protect turned into armor. Privacy became a survival skill. I smiled, I worked, I showed up for people, and I learned how to adjust my mask so it stayed in place even on the heaviest days. I wanted to be known for my hustle, my humor, my heart—not for the letters in my chart.

People often think secrecy is about shame; sometimes it's about stewardship. I didn't want the fragile, pitying looks or the slow, careful questions. I didn't want to be measured against a diagnosis. I didn't want to become the cautionary tale in someone else's mouth. MS made me ten times more private than I had ever been. The world already misreads what it cannot see; I refused to become anyone's misunderstanding.

But here's the thing about truths we bury: they keep breathing. They keep knocking. They keep asking to be born.

The knocking grew louder after my divorce. I had walked through fire and crawled out still singing, even if the notes were raspy. There was a day—no confetti, no chorus—just me, a quiet room, and the slow recognition that something inside had shifted. I had gotten through something I once believed would break me. And suddenly, all the reasons I'd used to stay silent sounded small.

It wasn't only the divorce. The truth had been ripening for years. I'd met strangers at MS walks and seminars who would catch my hands in theirs and ask, "How are you doing this? What's your secret?" They'd listen while I explained my therapy routine, how long I'd been on the same medication, the way I measured my days by energy and grace rather than hours and tasks. Sometimes they'd hug me as if I'd lent them a little hope to tuck into their pockets. I didn't feel like a hero; I felt ordinary—and somehow that made it matter more. Ordinary people, ordinary days, living an extraordinary reality: waking up sick and choosing to keep living.

The truth is, I didn't want to be anyone's symbol. I didn't want to be "the girl with MS who still smiles." I wanted to be Daneshia who just lives. But God and purpose can be persistent. My friends started saying what my own spirit had been whispering: "Tell your story." I could hear an old, careful voice inside me respond, "No. Not yet." Then another, bolder voice rose up with the insistence of dawn: "Now."

When I finally said yes, it surprised even me. Maybe because there wasn't one dramatic moment, no lightning bolt. It was more like a succession of small obediences. The MRI reports that kept returning dormant. The mornings I woke up heavier than sleep, but still folded the day into my hands like laundry and carried it. The faces I couldn't forget from those walks and seminars, people doing the impossible in bodies that felt uncooperative. The way my son watched me—curious, absorbing, quietly taking notes on what strength looks like when it's tired.

And then there was freedom tugging the hem of my shirt. I could feel it. Freedom has a sound; it rustles. It hums. It said: "There's a life on the other side of this silence."

I won't pretend I wasn't afraid. I'm afraid every day. MS is an invitation to uncertainty that never RSVP's—she just shows up and sits on your chest. One day you're laughing in the car; the next you wake with half your scalp numb and the world slightly tilted. Symptoms move like weather: insomnia that refuses to loosen its grip, speech that trips on its way out of your mouth, bowels that act like strangers, urgency that sends you to the bathroom again and again, tremors that hum beneath the skin, the eerie hug that clamps your midsection and convinces your body it's sprinting toward a heart attack. There's foot drop, when walking becomes negotiation; blurred vision and double vision, when up and down disagree; three and a half weeks of numbness in a limb that used to obey. I have woken into days that began with a symptom I couldn't see and couldn't hide—only endure. I've been on disability when the body said "Not today." Three times, in fact.

Try explaining all of that to people who can't see it. Try explaining why "I'm tired" means something different to me than it does to them. Try explaining why Thursdays once belonged to fatigue because my injections were on Wednesdays. The day after felt like Mike Tyson had used me as a speed bag. People would joke—lighthearted, not malicious—and then, over time, they learned. They respected the invisible. That learning curve took years.

Maybe that's one of the most exhausting parts of an invisible illness: the education. The constant gentle teaching so people don't misread your silence, your pace, your no. I am grateful for the ones who listened. I am grateful for the ones who, when they invited me on a Thursday and I said, "That's my tired day," didn't push. There's dignity in being believed.

It took me a long time to extend that same dignity to myself. Privacy can be holy. It can also become a cage. Mine had started to feel like both. Writing this book became the key.

At first, the words came slow, like unthawing. I would write and cry and write and laugh and write and breathe. Freedom became the loudest voice in the room. I could feel the weight lifting with each page. Healing didn't wait until the end—healing arrived in the middle, messy and unorganized, sitting beside me as I typed. That's what I wish more people understood: healing is motion. It's the decision to step forward while your knees still shake. It's not something earned after you've done everything "right." It's something that meets you while you're still choosing, afraid and stubborn and hopeful.

If you're newly diagnosed, here's what I want you to know: you can still build. It might take longer. You might need to build differently. But your life is not over; it's opening. Keep the degree on your list even if it stretches across a decade. Keep the dream in your mouth even if you can only whisper it. Keep the plans, and give yourself permission to rearrange them without apology. There are no gold stars for pretending you're not tired. There is honor in finishing—first, last, or steady in the middle.

Raising awareness matters because ignorance isolates. Before MS, I had heard the term and still didn't really know what it meant. MS is everywhere and nowhere: an illness too quiet to be seen, too loud to be ignored. So many people don't know what it is. I didn't, until it lived with me. So much of the stigma grows out of that emptiness—people fill the gap with fear. The story we tell about an illness determines how we treat the people who have it.

I learned awareness by doing. I read. I listened. I showed up. I walked—literally—at MS Walks with Team Tang (yes, like the orange drink, because our color is orange and I always liked to make things a little fun). Family and friends showed up in shirts and smiles, and we made the invisible visible for a day. I sat in rooms at seminars with folks who didn't always look like me and folks who did, and every time I spoke my truth, I was met with hands and questions and astonishment. Some people couldn't believe I had a child, that I still pursued acting and modeling, that I worked and went to school and took care of my mother and kept a house humming and didn't look like the illness that lived inside me. Their wonder used to make me uneasy. Now, I accept it as testimony.

I have no miracle routine to sell you. I've been on the same medicine for nearly twenty years. I am not the perfect exerciser with the perfect diet; I am a woman who prays, stretches, goes to StretchLab twice a month when I can, and pays attention to her body. I check in with a therapist when my mind needs tending, because muscles aren't the only thing that stiffen under pressure. I lean into music, the oldest therapy I know. And I keep a village—people who spoon-fed me courage when I forgot how to eat it by myself.

Awareness also means correcting what's wrong. MS is not a single story. Some of us walk, some of us don't. Some of us look "fine" and live with pain that would make others weep. Some of us are parents. Some of us are married. Some of us are single and thriving. None of those states makes us more or less "legitimate." Don't challenge an MS warrior's account of their body. Believe us the first time. If we say we're tired, that fatigue is a biology, not a character flaw. If we cancel, it's protection, not disrespect. If we slow down, it's wisdom, not weakness.

For a long time, the thought of telling my story terrified me. I worried about how it would be received, about offending my ex, about protecting my family from the intimacy of my truth. I worried about how I'd be seen once the mask came off. And yet, I kept writing. Anxiety and joy danced together across the page. Relief arrived in ripples. Pride, the good kind—the kind that says, "Look at God, and then look at what He carried me through"—rose in my chest.

People think you wait to write your story until the storm clears. But storms return. Healing has levels. I learned that the hard way. Even after I started writing, the old fear came back around the block to see if it could still find the front door. It's normal. I took the fear by the hand and brought it with me anyway.

The question I ask myself now is the one I hope this book answers for someone else: *If not now, when? If not you, who?*

Every year the MRIs returned with that word "dormant," and I felt like God was tapping my shoulder. Not to say I was cured, but to say I was carried. The appointments stitched a quiet testimony: *You're still here. Now do something with that.* I had spent so much time being every-one else's cheerleader that I forgot how to clap for myself. Writing this book reminded me. I am not the "despite." I am the "and." I have MS and I mother. I have MS and I create. I have MS and I laugh. I have MS and I rest.

If there's one person I'm writing for beyond myself, it's my son. I want him to understand the kind of strength that doesn't always look loud. I want him to look back and say, "My mother did not quit." When he's grown and leafs through these pages, I want him to hear me telling him what I tell him with my life: you can do hard things with grace. You can follow through at your pace. You can be both tender and unbreakable. You can love and set boundaries. You can honor your limits without abandoning your dreams.

And to the MS community—my people before we've even met—if I could sign up to be a face that says "It's possible," I would do it without a check. Free 99, as I like to joke, because purpose pays in a currency I can't deposit. If God trusts me with a platform, then I'm going to stand on it and tell the truth. Use my picture on a therapy brochure. Put my words in a magazine. Let me stand at a podium or on a stage and say, "I'm here. I'm living well. It's not easy. But it's possible."

Choosing to share my story has been less a reveal than a release. I did not land on healing like a destination; healing broke in like light under a door I finally opened. I won't pretend the vulnerability is gone. I still feel the tremble. But now the tremble feels like a prelude, not a warning.

If you are reading this and you've been hiding—your diagnosis, your divorce, your grief, your fear—consider this permission to let a little light in. Not because you owe the world your pain, but because hiding can turn pain into identity. Speaking can turn it into testimony.

I used to say, "Why me?" Now I say, "Why not me?" Not as resignation, but as calling. I have always worn many hats. I used to wonder if that was scattered. Now I see it as design. Each role trained me to carry this one: storyteller. Not because my story is perfect, but because it is true. Because it is ordinary and holy and stubbornly hopeful. Because it may invite someone else to breathe easier, to put down the shame, to trade the mask for mercy.

When I picture the end of this book, I don't see the period. I see a door swinging open. I see a room filling with people who begin to say out loud what they used to only whisper. I see women divorcing what diminishes them, parents setting down guilt, men learning how to ask for help, warriors with invisible battles finally being believed. I see my mother reading these pages and lifting her chin a little higher. I see my son, older now, pointing to a sentence with a smile that says, "That's my mama."

What do I hope you carry from this chapter? That silence can be sacred, but truth sets a table where you can finally eat. That privacy can be a protective blanket, but it can also be a weight. That telling your story won't always bring applause; sometimes it brings peace. And peace is the kind of wealth that pays your rent in the midnight hour.

If you are newly diagnosed: you are not broken. You are not late. You are not less-than. You're learning a new language for your body, and it will take time to become fluent. You will overdo it sometimes, and then you will learn to rest without apology. You will grieve the old ease, and then you will discover a new rhythm that carries its own beauty.

Let people help. Keep a therapist in your corner. Stretch. Pray. Sing. Find your "Thursday rules" and honor them. Say no without footnotes. Celebrate small wins like they are graduations—because some days, they are.

If you love someone with MS: believe them the first time. Don't argue with their limits or try to bargain with their fatigue. Respect the cancellations. Learn the language of invisible battles. Ask how to help, and be prepared for the answer to change.

And if you're me—if you're the me I used to be, with a book inside your chest and a fear inside your throat—start anyway. The words will teach you how to hold them. The page can take your weight. Freedom hums on the other side.

I think about all the times I almost didn't tell this story. Then I remember the faces at the walks, the women who squeezed my hands, the men who asked about medications and diets, the caregivers who wanted to know how to keep loving someone whose body shifts like weather. I remember the friends who nudged me toward the microphone, the colleagues who said, "You're not crazy for feeling scared; you're courageous for doing it anyway." I remember God's quiet insistence: *Now.*

So here it is—my silent battle, spoken. Not for spectacle, but for solidarity. Not to be exceptional, but to be honest. Not to be seen as strong, but to remind you that strength is a posture, not a performance.

I am living well with MS. I am a mother. I am a daughter. I am a sister. I am a friend. I am a woman who learned how to replace apology with authority, who learned that choosing herself is not betrayal but stewardship, who learned that healing has layers and love has limits and faith has legs.

This is not the end of my story; it's the end of my silence. And that, more than anything, is the victory I wanted.

Your Silent Battle Reflections:

1. What specific moment made you think, "It's time to tell my truth," and why?

2. If fear is present, what is it trying to protect you from—and what is it costing you?

3. How will you measure success as you share your story—by applause, or by peace?

4. Which practices keep you steady (faith, therapy, stretching, music, community), and how can you formalize them into a routine?

5. What is one concrete step you will take in the next 48 hours to move your truth forward?

Chapter 10

NEW BEGINNINGS

Life After Divorce

I never walked down the aisle expecting to one day walk away. Divorce wasn't in my plans, wasn't on my vision board, wasn't a part of the fairy tale I thought I was building. But life has a way of breaking us open and reshaping us into who we're meant to be.

When the papers were finalized, it was both an ending and a beginning. I remember sitting in the silence of my apartment one night, papers signed, the air heavy but still. The marriage was over. All the fighting, all the tears, all the years of trying to hold together what was already broken—it was done. And for the first time in years, I could hear myself think.

In that quiet, I realized something: I had survived.

Not just the divorce, but the years of silent battles—MS, caregiving, motherhood, heartbreak. I had survived them all. And survival wasn't the same as living, but it was the first step.

What surprised me most was what came next. I never could have imagined that the very illness I once thought would destroy me would become the platform that opened doors I never knew existed.

I had always loved theater. I went to school for it. I dreamed of stages and cameras and scripts with my name on them. For years, MS felt like it stole that dream from me. But after the divorce, something shifted. I began writing—not scripts for plays, not lines for auditions, but my story. My truth. At first, it was just journaling, just letting the pain and confusion bleed onto the page. But the more I wrote, the more I realized that my story wasn't just mine. It belonged to every woman who ever stayed silent. To every person living with an invisible illness. To every mother who gave until she had nothing left.

That's when *Silent Battles* was born.

Writing this book was never on my bucket list. I never thought I'd be an author, let alone someone writing about MS. I thought MS would keep me from living, not lead me into a new kind of life. Yet here I was, pouring my battles onto the page, and finding power in every word.

It was terrifying at first. To share what I had hidden for so long. To say out loud, "Yes, I have MS. Yes, I struggled in my marriage. Yes, I almost lost myself." But it was also freeing. The more I shared, the lighter I felt. Like I was pulling off layers of shame and fear I had carried for years.

And then the most unexpected thing happened. Opportunities started opening. Speaking engagements. Interviews. Even the chance to create a short documentary about my journey. Me—on camera, not just acting in a role, but telling my truth.

I remember shaking my head in disbelief. Theater had been my first love, but here was life giving me a second chance at it. Not in the way I had imagined, but in a way that felt deeper and more purposeful. This time, it wasn't about applause. It was about impact.

The milestones came one after another. Publishing my first book. Sharing my story on podcasts and radio. Standing on stages as a motivational speaker. Producing my first short film. Collaborating with people who believed in me, who saw the power of my testimony.

And the biggest milestone of all? Realizing I was stronger than I ever thought.

I used to think strength was about holding everything together—keeping the marriage intact, keeping the house clean, keeping the mask on so no one knew I was breaking. But real strength, I've learned, is in the breaking. It's in letting go of what's killing you. It's in standing up after the storm and saying, "I'm still here."

Three months after my divorce was finalized, I remember sitting in my car after a speaking event. I had just told a room full of people about my journey with MS, my divorce, my survival. And instead of pity, they clapped. They hugged me. They thanked me for sharing. One woman whispered, "Because of you, I don't feel so alone anymore."

I sat in my car and cried, but they were not tears of sorrow. They were tears of realization. I thought, *God, I'm stronger than I ever imagined. And this pain—it wasn't wasted.*

Managing MS & Building a New Life

Living with MS has always meant walking a fine line. Some days my body cooperates; some days it betrays me. After the divorce, that balancing act became even more important. I wasn't just managing MS anymore. I was managing MS as a single mom, as a daughter caring for a mother with Parkinson's, as a woman rebuilding a life from the ground up.

At first, I was terrified. I didn't know if I could do it. There were mornings I didn't want to get out of bed, when fatigue felt like chains around my body. But then I'd hear my son's voice—his laughter, his little footsteps—and I knew I had to rise.

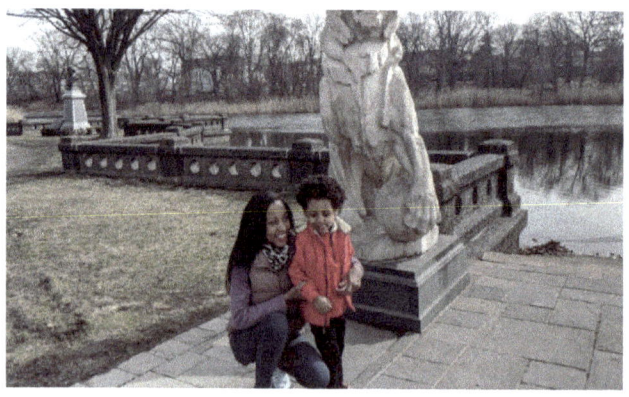

One thing I learned quickly: self-care wasn't optional. It was survival.

I developed routines that became my lifelines. Stretching at Stretch Lab twice a month, letting professionals help my body release the tension MS tried to hold hostage. Praying first thing in the morning and last thing at night, even if the prayers were just whispered sighs of "God, help me." Listening to music every day—gospel to lift me, R&B to remind me of love, even upbeat songs to make me dance in the kitchen with my son.

Therapy also became part of my healing. For years, I thought therapy was a weakness, a sign that I couldn't handle life. But now I see it as one of the strongest things I could do. Therapy gave me tools, gave me perspective, gave me permission to release the guilt I carried. It taught me to set boundaries, to say no without apology, to see myself not just as a caregiver but as a woman who deserved care too.

And I learned to ask for help. That was new for me. I used to wear independence like a badge of honor. I thought asking for help meant weakness. But MS humbled me. Divorce humbled me. Now I know that leaning on my village—friends, siblings, even my son in his small ways—is not weakness. It's wisdom.

Daily life is still a juggle. There are flare-ups, days when fatigue or numbness creeps in. But I no longer fight against the reality of MS. I flow with it. I pace myself. I forgive myself for not being able to do everything. I celebrate the small victories, like making it through the day without collapsing, like cooking dinner after a long day, like tucking my son in with a smile instead of tears.

MS didn't go away, but I no longer see it as my enemy. It's a part of my story, yes. But it's not the whole story.

Inner Strength & Lessons Learned

Heartbreak taught me resilience. Divorce taught me courage. MS taught me faith.

Looking back, I see qualities in myself I never fully recognized before. I see endurance—the kind that wakes up every day knowing the battle isn't over but fights anyway. I see empathy—because living with silent battles has made me softer toward others, more patient with their struggles. I see worthiness—because I finally believe I deserve love, respect, and joy, not just survival.

Heartbreak has a way of stripping you bare. For a long time, I thought it had taken everything from me. But in reality, it carved out space for new things: space for self-love, for independence, for joy that doesn't depend on anyone else.

One of the biggest lessons I've learned is that two good people can still be wrong for each other. Divorce doesn't always mean someone was a villain. Sometimes it just means the puzzle pieces don't fit. And that's okay.

I also learned the power of starting over. At first, starting over felt like punishment. But now I see it as a gift. A chance to rebuild, not from where I was, but from where I am now—with more wisdom, more faith, more clarity.

And perhaps the most important lesson: self-care is survival. If I don't fill my own cup, I can't pour into anyone else—not my son, not my mother, not my career. Choosing myself is not selfish. It's necessary.

Insights for Others

If there's one message I want to leave with anyone reading this, it's this: you are stronger than you think.

I know what it feels like to be broken. To cry in the shower so no one hears. To lie in bed and wonder how you'll face another day. To feel like illness, divorce, or loss has stolen your future.

But hear me: your story doesn't end there.

If God put you to it, He will see you through it. If you are breathing, there is still purpose in you. The battles you fight silently, the tears you cry in the dark—they are shaping you into someone stronger, someone wiser, someone who will one day look back and say, "I made it."

Don't ignore your red flags. Don't lose yourself trying to save someone else. Don't think that your worth is tied to being a wife, a mother, or anything else. You are worthy simply because you exist.

If my younger self—the scared, freshly divorced woman who thought her life was over—could see me now, she would be proud. Proud that I no longer people-please. Proud that I say no without guilt. Proud that I no longer shrink to make others comfortable. Proud that I stand, unapologetically, in my truth.

Divorce wasn't in my plan, but freedom was. MS wasn't in my plan, but purpose was. Heartbreak wasn't in my plan, but healing was.

And now, as I look ahead, I see not just battles, but victories. Not just endings, but beginnings.

This is my new chapter. My new beginning. My proof that broken things can be rebuilt, and sometimes, they come back even stronger.

Your Silent Battle Reflections:

1. What specific moment made you think, "It's time to tell my truth," and why?

2. If fear is present, what is it trying to protect you from—and what is it costing you? If not now, when?

3. What is one concrete step you will take in the next 48 hours to move your truth forward?

4. practices keep you steady (faith, therapy, stretching, music, community), and how can you formalize them into a routine?

5. What small win can you celebrate this week as evidence that your silence is ending?

Why Not Me?
AFFIRMATIONS

Read them aloud. Swap "I" for 'You' when you need to cheer on someone you love.

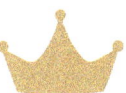

I am not my diagnosis. I am the author of my next page.

I carry what's heavy without it carry me.

I choose myself without apology, so I can love others with integrity.

My body's limits are not my spirit's limits.

Rest is sacred. Boundaries are love. No is a full sentence.

I honor small wins; they are bricks in my cathedral.

Fear can ride in the car, but it doesn't touch the wheel.

I am allowed to be brand-new after the storm.

A BENEDICTION FOR THE UNMASKED

May the truth you've spoken
make room for the life you deserve.

May your yes be aligned and
your no be holy.

May every flare, setback, or plot
twist remind you that grace is mobile.

May you find the people who hear you
the first time, hold your hand the
second, and fight beside you the third.

And when doubt whispers, *'Why you?'*,
may your spirit answer, *'Why not me?
I was built for this.*

THE READER'S PLEDGE

(Sign it, date it, tuck it in your book.)

I will treat my body as a home,
not a battlefield.

I will ask for help before the
breaking point.

I will celebrate progress over perfection.

I will speak to myself the way I would
speak to someone I love.

I will choose one brave action each week
that moves my life forward.

Signature: _____

Date: _____

A 7-Day UnMask Practice

Short, doable, MS-friendly — repeat as needed.

Day 1–Name it. Write one paragraph beginning with: *"The truth I've been hiding is..."*

Day 2–Body check. 5 minutes of gentle stretching or a short walk; note energy before/after.

Day 3–Boundary breath. Inhale: *"My needs matter."* Exhale: "I honor them." 3 minutes.

Day 4–One ask. Request support (ride, meal, childcare, listening ear). Receive it.

Day 5–Joy micro-dose. 10 minutes of music that lifts you; dance if you can, sway f you can't.

Day 6–Gratitude in detail. List three small wins with specifics (what you did, how it felt).

Day 7–Share your truth. Tell one trusted person what you're carrying and what helps.

For Anyone Facing MS (or Any Silent Battle)

You are not behind.

You're on a custom timeline.Fatigue is real; so is your permission to stop.

Track your patterns, protect your best hours, and make rest part of the
plan, not the reward.

Community is medicine. Find your people.

Keep the ones who believe you.

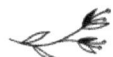

A Final Word from Daneshia

If this book found you in the dark, I hope it leaves you with a lit match
and a map. I wrote these pages to remind you and myself that surviving
isn't the whole story. We are allowed to rebuild, to reinvent, to rejoice. We
are allowed to be more than patients, partners, or parents. We are whole
people with holy futures. When the next hard day comes (and it will),
put your hand on your heart and repeat: "I am still here. And 'here' is
enough to begin again."

Closing Prayer for Silent Battles

Heavenly Father,

We thank You for the gift of life, for the strength that rises in us even when our bodies feel weak, and for the light that shines in the darkest corners of our journeys. Thank You for carrying us through battles that felt unbearable and for reminding us that we are never fighting alone.

Lord, I lift up every reader who holds this book in their hands. May these words breathe healing into their hearts, courage into their spirits, and hope into their futures. Remind them that their scars are not signs of defeat, but proof of survival. Teach them that their story has power, their pain has purpose, and their voice deserves to be heard.

Father, surround them with a community that uplifts and believes them. Give them peace on the hard days, rest for their weary souls, and joy that bubbles up even in the face of trials. Help them to remember that they are fearfully and wonderfully made, chosen and equipped for such a time as this.

And when life feels overwhelming, whisper to them the truth: "You are stronger than you think, braver than you believe, and loved more than you know."

May they leave these pages with renewed faith, unshakable resilience, and the boldness to walk in their truth unmasked.

In Jesus' mighty name, Amen.

Love you all,
Daneshia

Appendix

A. Resources for Individuals Dealing with MS

Living with Multiple Sclerosis (MS) can feel overwhelming, but you are not alone. The following organizations, communities, and resources provide education, support, and advocacy for individuals and families impacted by MS:

National Multiple Sclerosis Society (NMSS) – www.nationalmssociety.org

Offers comprehensive resources, including information on treatment, research updates, local chapters, fundraising walks, and peer support groups.

MS Foundation (MSF) – www.msfocus.org

Provides free educational materials, grants for medical equipment, and programs that support the daily needs of individuals living with MS.

MS International Federation (MSIF) – www.msif.org
A global network connecting people with MS across countries, sharing worldwide research, advocacy campaigns, and stories of resilience.

Can Do Multiple Sclerosis – www.cando-ms.org
Focuses on wellness education, lifestyle management, exercise, and nutrition guidance to help those with MS live healthier, more empowered lives.

MS Connection Program (through NMSS) – A peer-to-peer and online community offering support groups, mentor programs, and shared experiences for patients and caregivers.

Local Hospitals & MS Centers – Many regions have dedicated MS clinics or neurology departments offering personalized care, specialists, and support services.

Tip: Keep a "wellness team" — neurologist, primary care doctor, mental health professional, physical therapist, and support network — to help manage MS holistically.

B. Raising Awareness: Why It Matters

MS is often called an "invisible illness." Symptoms like fatigue, pain, brain fog, or numbness may not be visible to the outside world, which can make individuals feel unseen or misunderstood. Raising awareness helps bridge that gap.

Breaking the Silence: Sharing personal stories, whether through books, blogs, or conversations, helps others understand the realities of MS. It transforms invisible battles into visible truths.

Advocacy for Research and Treatment: The more people know about MS, the greater the push for research funding, better treatment options, and ultimately, a cure. Every voice raised adds power to this movement.

Fighting Stigma: Awareness challenges stereotypes that people with MS are "lazy" or "weak." It brings visibility to the unpredictable and exhausting nature of the disease.

Building Community: Campaigns such as MS Awareness Month (March) and events like Walk MS and Bike MS unite communities worldwide. These moments create solidarity and show those living with MS that they are never fighting alone.

Final Word in the Appendix

If you are reading this and living with MS or loving someone who does, then please know that your journey matters. Every story shared adds light. Every conversation creates change. And every step forward, no matter how small, is an act of courage.

Together, we fight not just for treatment but for understanding, empathy, and hope. Because we may have MS, but MS does not have us.

About the Author

Daneshia "This Is Me" Drakeford:

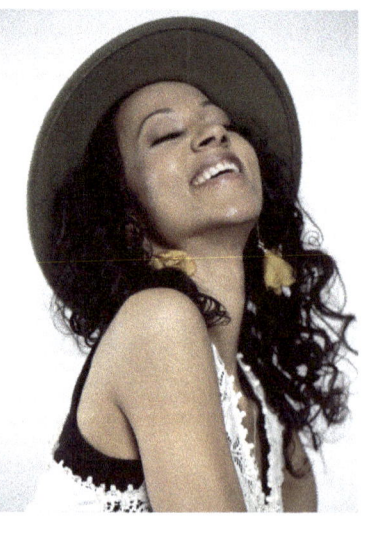

Daneshia Drakeford is a woman of resilience, faith, and courage. Diagnosed with Multiple Sclerosis in her twenties, she has spent nearly two decades fighting a battle few could see. For years, she carried her illness in silence, determined to push through school, work, motherhood, marriage, and caregiving without letting the world see her struggle. What once was her secret eventually became her testimony, a story she now shares with authenticity to inspire others.

Born and raised in New Brunswick, New Jersey, Daneshia has lived most of her life in the city that shaped her values of perseverance, family, and hard work. She worked for more than 25 years in customer service at Home Depot while also pursuing her first love of acting. A theatre student at Middlesex County College, she honed her craft on stage and screen, balancing her career, education, and health with an unshakable determination.

In her debut memoir *Silent Battles* (published by Jacinth Media Productions, available soon on Amazon Books, Barnes & Noble, and Walmart), Daneshia reveals the private struggles she once tried to keep hidden: a multiple sclerosis diagnosis, the weight of caregiving, the heartbreak of financial collapse, and the miraculous birth of her son against all medical odds.

After years of carrying these battles alone, she chose to reclaim her story. "I reached a point where I was no longer ashamed of my diagnosis or my journey," she shares. "This book is my way of standing in my truth and saying, 'This is me.'"

With *Silent Battles*, Daneshia delivers a powerful message of hope, faith, and resilience. She wants readers to know they are not alone, even when life's toughest trials feel invisible to the world. She sheds light on the unseen toll of MS, reminding audiences that strength often lives in the places no one can see. Her story highlights moments of fearless decision-making: defying doctors who told her not to have children, balancing motherhood with a chronic illness, rediscovering herself as a woman, and courageously rebuilding her acting career.

As she steps into this new chapter, Daneshia envisions expanding her advocacy through MS walks, seminars, and community outreach.

With dreams of becoming the face for MS awareness and even founding her own nonprofit, she is committed to using her platform to inspire, educate, and empower others.

Above all, Daneshia is a devoted mother, daughter, sister, and friend whose resilience shines through every role she carries. Her journey reminds us that illness does not define identity, and that even in the face of adversity, you can rise stronger, live boldly, and transform silent battles into powerful testimonies of survival.

Acknowledgements

Writing *Silent Battles* has been one of the hardest and most healing journeys of my life, and I could not have done it without the incredible people God placed in my corner. Each of you has poured into me in ways that became part of this book, and I am forever grateful.

To **Danny Collins**—thank you for always showing up with both hands and heart. From helping me with home projects to giving me honest, unfiltered feedback on this book, you've pushed me toward greatness. You never let me settle, and you reminded me that excellence is always worth fighting for.

To **Lanier "Wes" Westmoreland**—your wisdom, wit, and encouragement have been a gift since the day we met in acting class. You've always believed I was enough, even in the moments I doubted myself. Because of you, I stretched further than I thought I could, even into filmmaking. Thank you for challenging me and reminding me not to play small.

To **Jacinth Headlam**—my coach, my sissy pooh, and my friend. From acting to writing, from faith to motherhood, you've been there with guidance, encouragement, and love. You've poured life into me when I felt empty, and you've believed in this book just as much as I did. I couldn't have asked for a more genuine soul in my corner.

To **Assenka Oksiloff**, my mentor—thank you for your honesty and wisdom. You never sugarcoated the truth, but you always spoke it with love. You helped me see things from new perspectives, third lens, and encouraged me to grow beyond my comfort zone.

To **Lisa Daily-Winfrey**, my friend and stylist—you've done so much more than make me look good. Sitting in your chair was therapy. Thank you for the conversations about life, marriage, motherhood, and dreams, and for always sending me out into the world looking and feeling my absolute best.

To **Dr. Chandan Ahuja, DMD**—thank you for being such a huge part of bringing my *Silent Battles* documentary to life. Opening your office doors to us and supporting me in such a practical, tangible way was a blessing I'll never forget.

To my **Home Depot family**—thank you for the love, encouragement, and support you've shown me throughout this journey. You have been part of my story since the beginning, and I carry your support with me in everything I do.

To my **doctors and medical team**—thank you for walking this unpredictable road with me. Your dedication, care, and compassion have carried me through some of the hardest days.

And finally, to my **family and friends**—you've been my anchor. Every prayer, every word of encouragement, every time you stood by me when I felt like I was fighting alone—it mattered. You reminded me I was never truly alone.

This book is my testimony, but it's also a reflection of the village that carried me through the silence. Thank you for believing in me, for loving me through the storms, and for giving me the courage to share my truth with the world.

Notes

www.ingramcontent.com/pod-product-compliance
Lightning Source LLC
Chambersburg PA
CBHW051219120626
46547CB00013B/1418